W9-CUI-434

Time-Life
   Successful parenting: Food and
your child. By the editors of Time-
Life Books.   Time-Life Books, 1988.
   144 p. col. illus., col. photos.
   Bibliography: p. 138-139.

1. Children - Nutrition. 2.
Nutrition. I. Title. II. Title:
Food and your child.

Food and Your Child

By the Editors of Time-Life Books

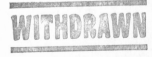
Alexandria, Virginia

TIME®
LIFE
BOOKS

Time-Life Books Inc.
is a wholly owned subsidiary of

Time Incorporated

FOUNDER: Henry R. Luce 1898-1967

Editor-in-Chief: Jason McManus
Chairman and Chief Executive Officer:
J. Richard Munro
President and Chief Operating Officer:
N. J. Nicholas, Jr.
Editorial Editor: Ray Cave
Executive Vice President, Books: Kelso F. Sutton
Vice President, Books: George Artandi

Time-Life Books Inc.

EDITOR: George Constable
Executive Editor: Ellen Phillips
Director of Design: Louis Klein
Director of Editorial Resources: Phyllis K. Wise
Editorial Board: Russell B. Adams, Jr., Dale M.
Brown, Roberta Conlan, Thomas H. Flaherty, Lee
Hassig, Donia Ann Steele, Rosalind Stubenberg, Kit
van Tulleken, Henry Woodhead
Director of Photography and Research:
John Conrad Weiser
Assistant Director of Editorial Resources:
Elise Ritter Gibson

PRESIDENT: Christopher T. Linen
Chief Operating Officer: John M. Fahey, Jr.
Senior Vice Presidents: Robert M. DeSena,
James L. Mercer
Vice Presidents: Stephen L. Bair, Ralph J. Cuomo,
Neal Goff, Stephen L. Goldstein, Juanita T. James,
Hallett Johnson III, Carol Kaplan, Susan J.
Maruyama, Robert H. Smith, Paul R. Stewart,
Joseph J. Ward
Director of Production Services:
Robert J. Passantino

Library of Congress Cataloging in Publication Data
Food and your child.
  (Successful parenting)
  Bibliography: p.
  Includes index.
  1. Children—Nutrition. 2. Nutrition. 3. Food.
I. Time-Life Books. II. Series.
TX361.C5F66 1988   649'.3—dc19   87-26736
ISBN 0-8094-5945-0
ISBN 0-8094-5946-9 (lib. bdg.)

Successful Parenting

SERIES DIRECTOR: Dale M. Brown
Series Administrator: Norma E. Shaw
Editorial Staff for *Food and Your Child:*
Designer: Raymond Ripper
Picture Editor: Marion F. Briggs
Text Editors: Margery A. duMond, John Newton
Researchers: Myrna Traylor-Herndon (principal),
Charlotte Fullerton, Sydney Johnson, Fran Moshos,
Nancy C. Scott
Assistant Designer: Susan M. Gibas
Copy Coordinators: Marfé Ferguson, Ruth Baja
Williams
Picture Coordinator: Linda Yates
Editorial Assistant: Patricia D. Whiteford

Special Contributors: Amy Aldrich, Susan Perry,
Irene Rosenberg, Barbara Sause, Charles C. Smith,
David Thiemann (text); Barbara Cohn, Melva
Holloman, Ann Muñoz Furlong (research).

Editorial Operations
Copy Chief: Diane Ullius
Production: Celia Beattie
Library: Louise D. Forstall

Correspondents: Elisabeth Kraemer-Singh (Bonn);
Maria Vincenza Aloisi (Paris); Ann Natanson
(Rome).

First printing. Printed in U.S.A.

Published simultaneously in Canada.
School and library distribution by
Silver Burdett Company, Morristown,
New Jersey 07960.

TIME-LIFE is a trademark of Time
Incorporated U.S.A.

Other Publications:

MYSTERIES OF THE UNKNOWN
TIME FRAME
FIX IT YOURSELF
FITNESS, HEALTH & NUTRITION
HEALTHY HOME COOKING
UNDERSTANDING COMPUTERS
LIBRARY OF NATIONS
THE ENCHANTED WORLD
THE KODAK LIBRARY OF CREATIVE PHOTOGRAPHY
GREAT MEALS IN MINUTES
THE CIVIL WAR
PLANET EARTH
COLLECTOR'S LIBRARY OF THE CIVIL WAR
THE EPIC OF FLIGHT
THE GOOD COOK
WORLD WAR II
HOME REPAIR AND IMPROVEMENT
THE OLD WEST

For information on and a full description
of any of the Time-Life Books series listed
above, please call 1-800-621-7026 or write:
Reader Information
Time-Life Customer Service
P.O. Box C-32068
Richmond, Virginia 23261-2068

This volume is one of a series about raising children.

The Consultants

The General Consultant

Dr. Laurence Finberg is Professor and Chairman of the Department of Pediatrics in the School of Medicine at the State University of New York Health Science Center, Brooklyn. He also serves as Chief of Pediatrics at the university's two associated hospitals, Kings County Hospital and University Hospital, Brooklyn. He is a consultant to the World Health Organization, and chairs the American Academy of Pediatrics' Committee on Nutrition. He has authored or coauthored numerous professional articles on children's health and nutrition.

Special Consultants

Dr. Leann Lipps Birch, an internationally recognized authority on the development of children's eating patterns and food preferences, helped prepare the section on the social, emotional, and developmental aspects of children's mealtime behavior *(pages 6–35)*. Dr. Birch is Division Chair and Professor of Human Development and Nutritional Science, in the Division of Human Development and Family Ecology, at the University of Illinois at Urbana-Champaign. She also serves on the editorial board of the *Journal of Nutrition Education.*

Lisa Cherkasky, a graduate of the Culinary Institute of America, developed and styled all of the recipes *(pages 106–137)*. Ms. Cherkasky is an experienced restaurant chef and cooking-school instructor; she also served as a recipe developer and food stylist for the Time-Life cookbook series "Healthy Home Cooking."

Dr. Elliot S. Ellis, who contributed his expert opinion on the hyperactive child *(page 72)*, is Chief of the Division of Allergy and Clinical Immunology at The Nemours Children's Clinic in Jacksonville, Florida. He was for ten years Codirector of the Division of Allergy and Immunology at Children's Hospital of Buffalo, New York, and served twelve years as a professor in the Department of Pediatrics, State University of New York at Buffalo, including nine years as the department's chairman. Dr. Ellis is a past president of the American Academy of Allergy and Immunology, and is the author or coauthor of many professional articles on children's health.

Mary T. Goodwin assisted with the section on food activities to share with your child *(pages 82–97)* and in the section on preserving and storing foods *(pages 98–105)*. As Chief Nutritionist for Maryland's Montgomery County Health Department, Ms. Goodwin has established nationally recognized programs in public health and in nutrition education. A well-known advocate for food assistance programs to improve children's nutrition, Ms. Goodwin is coauthor, with Gerry Pollen, of *Creative Food Experiences for Children.*

Janet E. Tenney, a registered dietician, helped with the chapter on nutrition *(pages 36–63)* and assessed the nutritive value of the recipes *(pages 106–137)*. The Manager of Nutrition Programs for a major regional supermarket chain, Ms. Tenney holds a master's degree in human nutrition. She was the nutrition consultant for the Time-Life cookbook series "Healthy Home Cooking."

Contents

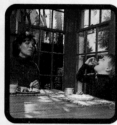
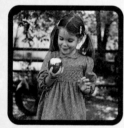
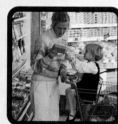

4

Good Times with Food   82

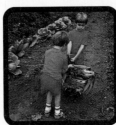

5

Practical Cooking for Hungry Youngsters   98

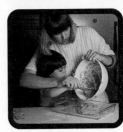

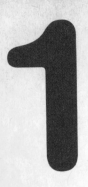

Your All-Important Role

Children are born to eat, and never does this seem more true than when your newborn signals you that he is hungry through his loud and lusty cry. With the first drink of formula or breast milk, your child begins a soothing relationship with food that will affect his future health and well-being. Developed early, positive attitudes toward nourishment and eating will greatly increase his chances of a good life. Negative attitudes can lead to obesity or other eating disorders. You will want, therefore, to make the feeding experience as good a one as it can be.

During your child's earliest years, as he matures from infant to kindergartner, you and he will share many profound changes in his eating behavior. He will enjoy a wider range of foods and develop new eating skills. He will progress from breast or bottle, to feeding himself with his fingers, to sitting up at the table with the grown-ups and manipulating spoon, fork, and knife. He will begin to learn the importance of table manners, mealtime conversation, and other customs connected with food. He will advance from total reliance on you for all his food to growing independence and control over his own eating. Above all, he will learn his most basic eating habits and food attitudes from you.

This chapter will guide you in the ways your feeding role will need to change as your child grows up. From nursing and spoon-feeding a baby, you will move on to supervising a toddler's messy self-feeding, then to enjoying the dinner-table prattle of a talkative preschooler. At every stage of development, you will meet both frustrations and rewards. Understanding the development of your child's relationship with food, and how it progresses along with his maturing social and emotional abilities, will help you anticipate and even enjoy each new kind of behavior. In turn, you will be giving him the chance to discover in eating a healthy source of physical and emotional gratification.

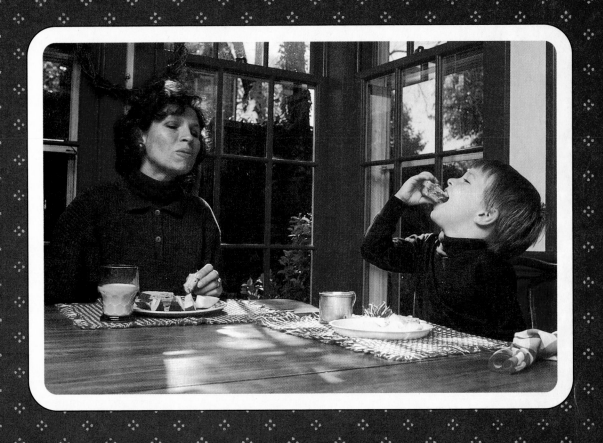

The Happiness of Eating

When you feed your child, much more is going on than the simple giving and taking of sustenance. Starting from her first feeding after birth, she begins to associate food with physical and emotional gratification. The comforts of being held, cuddled, cooed at, and caressed merge with the pleasures of sucking and tasting and filling up. In the infant's mind, food is love, and being well fed comes to mean being well cared for. As she advances from suckling to drinking from a cup and then to solid foods and self-feeding, eating and drinking continue to have great psychological significance.

For you as a parent, mealtime will also be emotionally important. In supplying food, you are providing survival itself, and your baby's utter dependence on you is one of the most heart-touching aspects of parenting. Perhaps the greatest challenge you will face as a parent is to relinquish this dependence, gradually and sensitively, as you help your child attain the autonomy she seeks.

With needs so great on both sides of the relationship, conflict may arise. The better you understand the dynamics involved, the better equipped you will be to deal positively with the difficult times and to enjoy the good times all the more.

The basis for attachment

A newborn's first sustained contact with another human being revolves largely around being fed. As you nurse or bottle-feed your baby in the months following birth, a natural, rhythmic communication ebbs and flows between you. Sometimes he will gaze up at you as he nurses; sometimes he will take a break from sucking to smile, or to explore you with his eyes and hands. In this way, feeding builds lasting attachment.

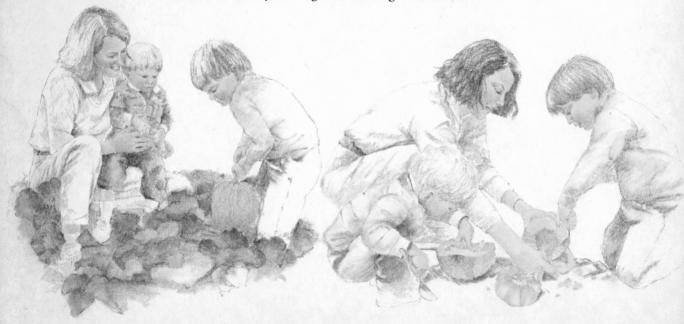

By giving your child love and attention along with breast or bottle, and recognizing his capacity to give you love and attention in return, you help him to form an important bond. In making each feeding a time of warmth, comfort, cuddling, and intimacy, you satisfy an emotional hunger that is as important as your baby's physical hunger for food. The attachment that grows between you, and the association between food and love that develops in the baby's mind, will be the basis for his feelings about food as he grows up.

Good eating and good feelings
The immediate connection between your child's food and her feelings is obvious — a hungry child tends to get cranky. This clear short-term connection between eating and feeling good is reflected in the long-term link between how children eat and how they feel about themselves. Being well nourished promotes not only physical health and growth but emotional well-being. Eating properly and feeling good physically make it easier for your child to develop the self-esteem she needs to become a happy, confident adult.

The many meanings of food
It is perfectly natural for food to take on, for both parents and children, other meanings beyond its nutritional value. Virtually every human culture invests certain foods with special significance. Some items are taboo, some are used in religious rituals, some become status symbols, and some are credited with healing powers. But in almost every household, food becomes a symbol of love. This symbolism is wholesome, if it helps you feel good about your nourishing and nurturing abilities. It is a

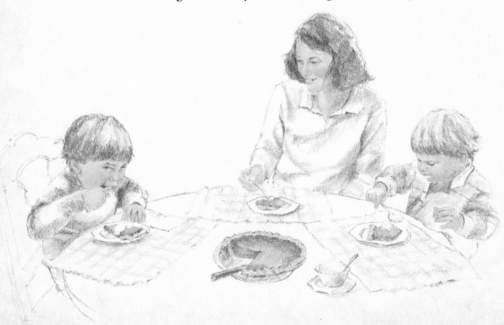

In their quest for a pumpkin pie, two boys and their mother savor a series of memorable activities, from harvesting the fruit on a sunny autumn day, to scraping out the seeds, to sharing the tasty pie at the family table. Learning where foods come from helps children feel a special sense of connectedness with the dishes that make up their meals.

problem, however, if you give food as your only means of giving love, if you regard your child's every refusal to eat as a rejection of you, or if you overfeed her in an effort to convince yourself that you are a good provider.

Hunger and appetite

The psychological aspects of eating are especially evident at family mealtimes, when parents' and children's enjoyment of each other's company is as life-giving as the food they eat together. The atmosphere you create is crucial; though nature will make your child hungry, it is up to you to stimulate his appetite so that he eats happily and well. Emotionally satisfying food experiences characterized by family sharing, warmth, and intimacy make any dish immensely more appealing.

The battle for good nutrition

You may sometimes find it hard not to force food on your child. Having her best nutritional interests at heart, you may be frustrated by her refusal to eat things you know are good for her. When she is still nursing or being spoon-fed, she may turn away from food you offer, or accept it and then spit it out. Once she is feeding herself *(charts, pages 11–17)*, she may anger you by playing with food or dumping it on the floor. Such behavior, though perfectly normal, can lead to serious conflict between you and your child if you do not see it as natural and something to expect from time to time. Regardless of how upset you may feel, do not permit your youngster to goad you into using such negative tactics as force, threats, or bribes to promote eating. If you respect her need to exercise some control over her own intake, and if you educate yourself about nutrition *(pages 38–44)* and share your knowledge with her in a positive and loving way, you can head off many mealtime battles. Indeed, you can avoid having her control you through her eating behavior.

You can begin your child's nutritional education at an early age. A two-year-old is capable of understanding the need to eat certain foods and avoid others. Your most powerful educational tool is your own example: If your youngster sees you choosing healthful snacks, eating varied, nutritious meals, and enjoying fresh fruit for dessert, he will do the same. To give your child a valuable sense of control over what he eats, offer him some choices when it comes to meal planning and let him help out on shopping trips. Making him feel involved in family menus will not eliminate mealtime outbursts altogether — some conflict about food is just part of growing up — but it will help you create the kind of atmosphere that fosters sound nutrition and good emotional health. ∴

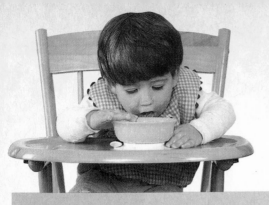

Onward and Upward with Food

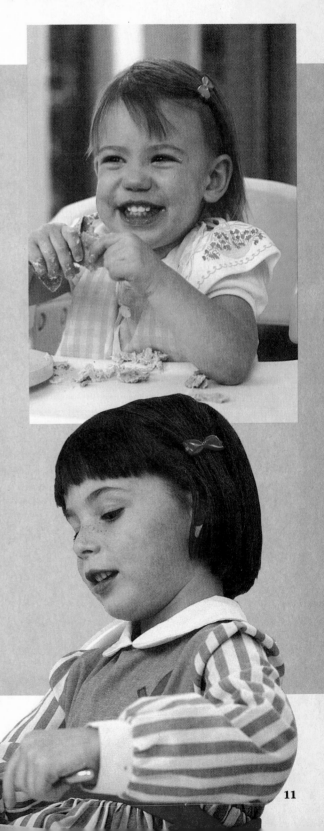

You will see many dramatic changes in your child's eating habits as she grows from infant into toddler and then preschooler. The better you understand the process, the more comfortable you will be with each phase along the way, and the more you can help your child acquire good eating habits.

The charts on the following pages trace a child's evolving relationship with food. The material is divided under three headings: Feeding Skills, Mealtime Behavior, and Appetite. Feeding Skills focuses on the developing motor and sensory abilities that increasingly allow the child to participate directly in feeding. Mealtime Behavior includes the ways he acts toward his food and the people around him while he is eating. Appetite concentrates on the child's capacity for food, as reflected in the number and size of the meals he can eat at different ages, shifts in his food preferences, and the ways he has of indicating that he is full. Each chart covers a separate period of childhood: infancy, from birth to one year; toddlerhood, ages one to three; and the preschool years, ages three to six.

These charts will help you know what to expect from your young one and may help calm some concerns about noisy or messy feeding. For example, the charts show that some behaviors, such as spitting out food or throwing it on the floor, possibly considered bratty or defiant in an older child, are normal acts of playfulness and food exploration in a baby. The five-month-old who is easily distracted during feedings is not trying to annoy — she is merely honing her perceptual skills of looking and listening. And you may find a toddler's resistance to being fed more tolerable, and a lot less frustrating, when you know it signals her new urge toward independence.

Bear in mind that charts like these are not inflexible timetables; the information set out here represents generalizations about how most children eat. You need not worry that your child is behind if she is slow in displaying some of the behaviors described. By the same token, she is not necessarily a prodigy if she is ahead of schedule in other areas. In eating, as in every aspect of her growth and development, each child is a unique individual. The purpose of these charts is to give you some averages you can use to anticipate and understand your child's approach to food.

Infants (Birth to 1 Year)

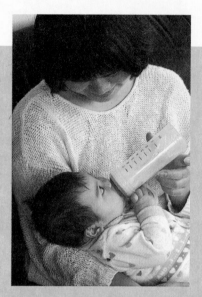

Feeding Skills

- At birth, baby cries to indicate hunger, responds to taste sensations, distinguishes among different tastes. Seeks food by "rooting" with the head, turning it methodically from side to side in search of the nipple.

- At birth, gets milk by licking the nipple rhythmically, swallows when liquid comes into mouth. Between 1 and 5 months, learns to coordinate sucking and swallowing with breathing.

- From birth, makes biting motion when gums are touched. By 4 to 6 months, can swallow strained or pureed foods. At 4 to 8 months, uses tongue to move food around in mouth. At 5 to 8 months, mouths and gums solid food. Around 6 months, learns normal biting, bites soft solid food. By 7 months, has less urge to suck, can take solid food at the beginning of a meal. By about 6 to 7 months, learns chewing, is ready to eat grown-up foods. Might have difficulty accepting such foods later if not introduced to them now. By 9 to 10 months, bites off proper size mouthful, chews easily.

- Around 6 months, shows interest in manipulating food with hands, closes palm around pieces of food, lifts them to face. At 7 to 8 months, does messy self-feeding, picking up pieces with thumb and first two fingers. By 11 months, is able to feed self using thumb and forefinger. Enjoys a feeling of accomplishment from this control of food.

- At 6 to 7 months, if has had experience with solid food, anticipates spoon-feeding with eagerness. By about 9 to 12 months, holds spoon. By 1 year wants to manage the spoon by himself — but is not always successful.

- At 6 to 8½ months, drinks from cup held by someone else, with lips in only approximate contact with rim, resulting in some dribbling. Between 7 and 9 months, notices cup being filled, makes eager sounds, opens mouth, reaches for cup with both hands. Around 9 months, holds cup by handle. At 10 to 12 months, tilts head as well as cup. Lip contact with rim improves, dribbling decreases.

Mealtime Behavior

- At 6 to 10 weeks, recognizes feeding position: begins sucking and mouthing when placed in typical feeding position. By 2 months, recognizes parent as a source of food. Around 3 months, looks at the face of mother or another caregiver when drinking, smiles and coos.

- Between 3½ and 4½ months, recognizes bottle on sight. At 4 to 5 months, pats bottle. At 4½ to 5½ months, touches bottle with both hands. Between 5½ and 9 months can hold bottle.

- By about 4 months, is readily distracted during feeding by sights, sounds, and other stimuli.

- Around 5 months, learns to manipulate feeding session by refusing to eat.

- By about 6 to 7 months, if already on solid foods, shows desire to be spoon-fed by reaching eagerly with head and mouth.

- At about 8 months, will reach for food, pound, and throw food, cup, and utensils.

- By 6 to 8 months, smears, pokes, and spits out food, not necessarily to reject it, but to explore it through smelling and handling. At about 12 months, removes food from mouth, looks at it, puts it back in.

- May start to wean self as early as 6 months; will sometimes signal readiness by pulling away from breast or bottle, showing interest in foods eaten by the rest of the family. However, signals of readiness may not appear until 2 or 3 years of age.

- By 1 year, may want to stand up at table and play.

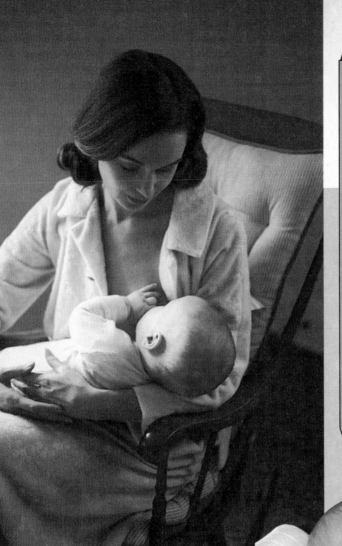

Appetite

- At birth, feeds six to twelve times a day at two- to four-hour intervals, drinking two to three ounces at a time. By 2 months, feeds five times a day, drinks up to thirty-five ounces daily, the equivalent of about four-and-a-half cups. At about 6 months, has four milk feedings and three meals a day. By 9 to 10 months, has three meals a day, with a fruit-juice snack in mid-afternoon. By 12 months, eats three meals a day, has a bottle after supper or at bedtime.

- At birth, indicates fullness and satisfaction by falling asleep with the nipple in mouth, or by giving up sucking and starting to play with the nipple. Around 4 to 6 months, uses whole body to announce fullness and desire to stop eating; signals include arching back, squirming, kicking, fussing, crying, throwing head back and twisting it from side to side. At around 10 months, shakes head no, turns head and purses lips, bites spoon or own tongue to express fullness. Between 10 and 12 months, indicates fullness by banging cup, passing it from hand to hand, biting its bottom, sticking fingers into cup or mouth, turning head or pursing lips.

- Around 4 to 6 months, accepts cereal and then fruit. Between 6 and 12 months, is increasingly interested in eating the same foods as other family members. As soon as solid foods are introduced, shows preference for some over others. At around 12 months, might decide that sweets are favorite.

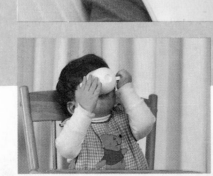

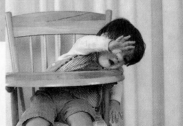

Toddlers (1-3 Years)

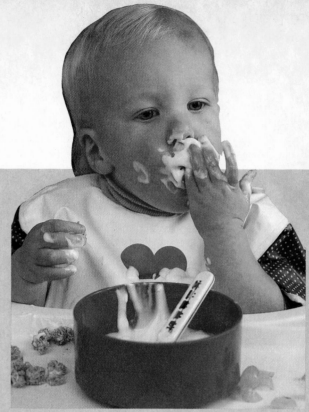

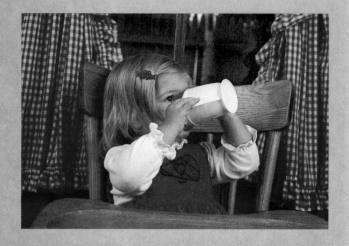

Feeding Skills

- Between 12 and 14 months, toddler wants to spoon-feed self, is not always successful. At 12 to 15 months, holds spoon in fist and brings it toward face, but often turns it over before it reaches mouth. By 18 months, grasps spoon in one hand; holds spoon to plate. Can hold spoon horizontally; has learned to raise elbow while lifting spoon to mouth and to turn spoon only after it is in mouth. May insist on eating a whole meal without help. At 21 months, can grasp spoon with thumb pressed parallel against side of handle. By 2 years, puts spoon in mouth correctly.

- Between 12 and 14 months, drinks from cup, using both hands; but still tilts head with cup. Between 12 and 18 months, gains more skill at drinking from cup; takes five or six swallows at a time, tilting cup only but often spilling contents. By 18 months, has good cup control, with little or no spilling. Between 20 and 30 months, drinks from small cup held in one hand.

- Between 12 and 14 months, chews well, but without mature chewing pattern. Between 15 and 18 months, probably has some molars and can chew tough foods with rotary jaw movement. About 18 to 24 months, chews entirely with rotary jaw action.

- By 15 months, is skillful at finger feeding.

- Around 23 to 25 months, can peel a banana and unwrap packaged foods.

- Around 28 months, can get food on fork and into mouth.

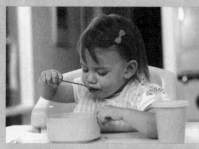

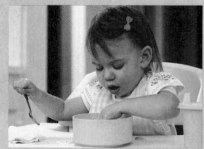

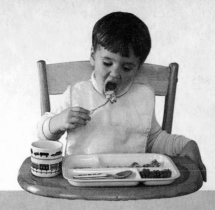

Mealtime Behavior

- Around 12 to 14 months, makes jabbering noises to express need for food.

- By 12 to 14 months, as walking and decision-making abilities confer increasing independence, may resist being fed, refuse to try new foods. Mealtime becomes an opportunity to test personal autonomy.

- Around 18 to 21 months, loves mealtime rituals, may insist on always using same bib, cup, spoon, or dish. May even reject a favorite food if rituals are violated.

- By 18 to 24 months, may voluntarily give up bottle or breast-feeding.

- At 19 to 23 months, plays with food, turning a cracker, for example, into a person or a car.

- Between 30 and 36 months, learns to use napkin.

- After 31 months, takes an interest in helping with the setting of the table.

Appetite

- By 1 year, needs three meals a day and two snacks of appropriate size, one in morning, one in afternoon.

- Between 12 and 18 months, may show declining appetite and refuse food as rapid growth spurt of first year tapers off. Teething may also reduce appetite.

- From 2 to 2½ years, as food preferences become more consistent, may demand familiar items and familiar brand names and express definite food preferences. May also become extremely fussy about diet, sometimes demanding one item repeatedly, only to drop it in favor of a new favorite. May reject many foods.

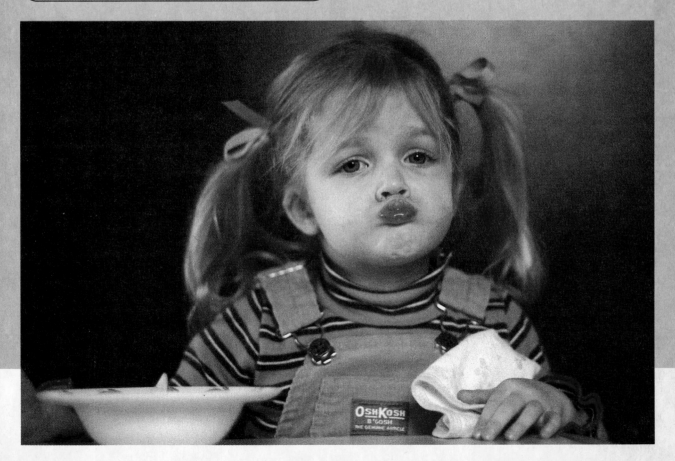

Preschoolers (3-6 Years)

Feeding Skills

- At 3 years, preschooler grasps spoon with thumb and index finger. By 4 years, feeds self with spoon held in adult fashion, between thumb and first two fingers.

- By 3 years, drinks from cup in adult fashion, using one hand to hold it by the handle.

- By 3 years, can pour liquids from small containers. By 3½ years, turns faucet on and off to fill a cup with water. By 4 years, pours from a pitcher into a cup, can carry the cup without spilling the contents. By 4 years, can prepare a bowl of cereal, pouring cereal and milk in appropriate amounts with little or no spilling.

- At 3 years, often demands a fork, makes a fist to hold it. By 4 years, holds it between thumb and first two fingers, uses it skillfully to pierce pieces of food and carry them to the mouth without dropping.

- Between 3 and 4 years, can use a knife to butter bread. At 5 years, may be able to cut food with a knife.

- By 4 years, serves self at the table, transferring food in appropriate portion sizes from serving dish to plate. Passes dishes to other family members.

Mealtime Behavior

- At 3 years, eats neatly, seldom asks for help with eating. Is ready to learn simple table manners; can be taught to keep mouth closed while chewing.

- At 3 years, can stay seated at the table for 10 to 15 minutes at a time. Enjoys eating at a small table with other children. May sit still longer and eat more in this situation than with the family.

- Between 3 and 4 years, can help with simple aspects of table clearing and cleanup after meals. By 4 years, is able to set the table.

- Between 3 and 4 years, may refuse to eat the food you prepare and demand, something else; may deliberately insist on having foods that are not in the house.

- Around 4 to 5 years, may use rude behavior at the table as an attention-getting device. May sometimes dominate dinner conversation.

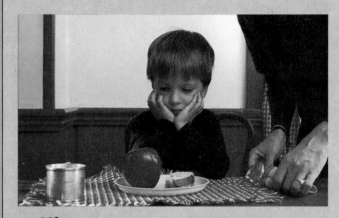

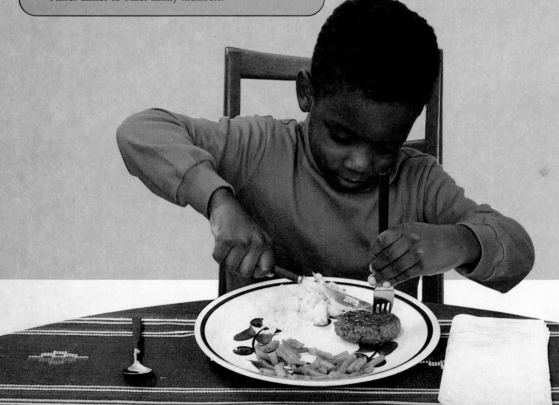

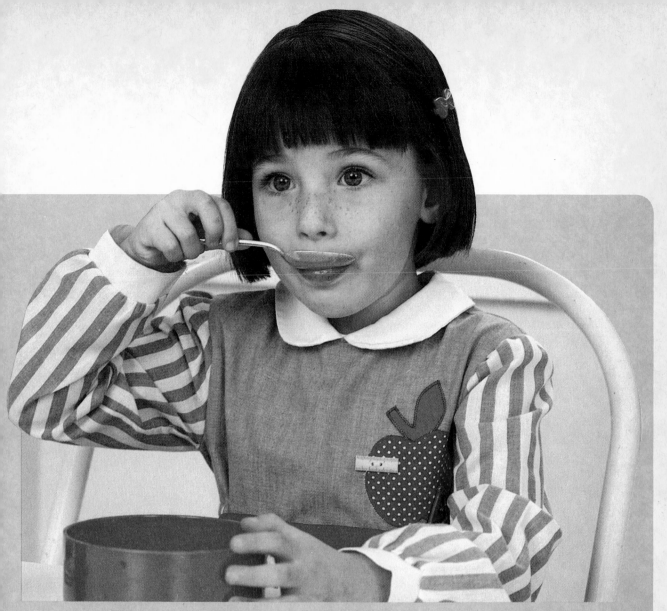

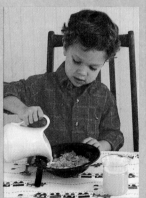

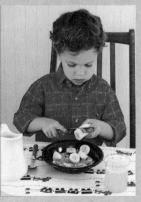

Appetite

- Needs three meals and two small snacks each day.

- By 3 years, often prefers foods that require extra chewing, such as raw vegetables and meat on the bone.

- Between 3 and 4 years, displays increasing willingness to try new foods and may accept some that were once rejected. By 5 years, may try new foods without complaining and beg for foods featured in TV commercials.

- Around 4 years, expresses many strong food preferences, tends to demand familiar items repeatedly; during meal preparation, may ask for special favorite. Sometimes has eating whims, stages hunger strikes.

- Between 4 and 5 years, may manifest declining appetite, finding play activities often more diverting than food.

- At 5 years, still prefers small portions of simple foods, may dislike two or more foods mixed together.

How Much and When?

Two common concerns of parents are how much to feed their children and when. No doubt questions have arisen in your own mind concerning such matters. What mealtimes should you establish? What should your snack policy be? How much food is enough? Feeding a nursing infant is relatively simple, but as the baby grows older, her eating habits will change, shaped by psychological and developmental factors, and you will have to keep up with them.

Mealtimes, regular but flexible

In mealtimes as in other daily events, youngsters thrive on stability and routine. Make an effort to be consistent, serving your child his meals at the same hours each day. His mealtimes, however, need not correspond to those of older members of the family. If you eat dinner at 6:00 P.M., but your child is hungry at 4:00 P.M, by all means feed him at that time, when he is ready to eat well, or tide him over with a snack.

The dangers of overfeeding

The problem of overeating often starts in infancy, when parents offer food every time the baby fusses. Babies do cry when they are hungry, but that is not the only cause, and parents who act as if it were may be paving the way for obesity and other eating problems. Older children who are made to eat more than they really want will soon learn to associate receiving food with oppressive authority, and refusal of food with their own personal autonomy. This pattern of thinking can lead in the teenage years to anorexia, bulimia, and other life-threatening eating disorders.

It is best to offer your youngster food without threats, bribes, cajolery, or pressure tactics. And avoid overfeeding her. Put modest portions on her plate. A 3-year-old needs only about half as much food as an adult, a 6-year-old only two-thirds as much. If your youngster dislikes what she has been given, do not disrupt your meal to prepare something special for her, and do not imagine that her health depends on her cleaning up her plate. If she chooses not to eat, she will more than likely survive until the next meal or snack.

Signals of satiety

When a nursing baby is satiated, she may stop sucking and fall asleep. A spoon-fed infant will turn her head away or spit food out. Older children will tell you one way or another when they are full. By letting your child stop when she indicates she is sated, you are telling her that you value her participation in the feeding process and respect her ability to take some control over her own eating.

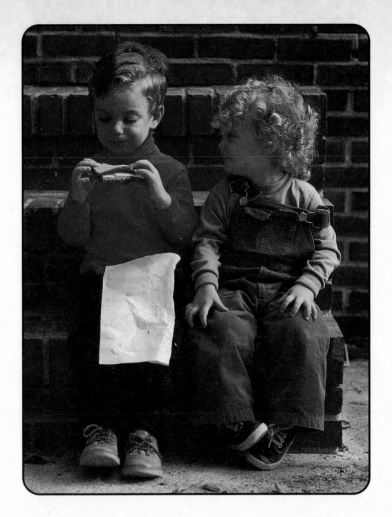

Between-meal snacks, bad and good

Parents often worry that eating between meals will harm a child by "spoiling his appetite," causing him to eat less than he needs at mealtimes. Obviously there is some truth to this notion; a child who consumes a handful of jellybeans just before dinner probably will not finish his meal. Some controlled snacking, however, makes nutritional sense. Because children have smaller stomachs than adults, they are better off eating in small installments throughout the day instead of relying on three large meals hours apart. You can make snacking a positive part of your child's diet if you watch the timing and content of his snacks. A reasonable schedule might allow one snack at midmorning, and one in the afternoon. Provide nutritious foods such as low-fat cheeses, bread and crackers, fruits, raw vegetables, milk, and juice. Downplay sugar, but remember that not all sweets are created equal. Oatmeal cookies are more nourishing than chocolate chips and contain fiber to boot; ice cream and pudding, though sugary, still offer the same protein and calcium found in unsweetened milk products. Well-chosen snacks can enhance your child's eating pleasure, as well as his health. ∴

Understanding Your Young One's Preferences

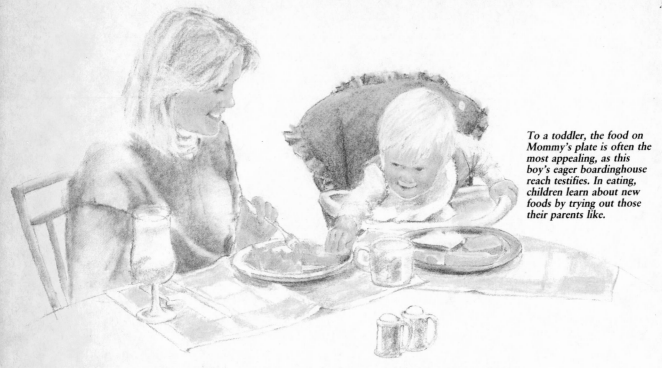

To a toddler, the food on Mommy's plate is often the most appealing, as this boy's eager boardinghouse reach testifies. In eating, children learn about new foods by trying out those their parents like.

In eating, as in so many other areas of her life, one of the greatest influences on your child's behavior will be the example you set. Whether you intend it or not, you are destined to be a primary role model in her earliest years. If you wish to teach your child to eat a nutritious diet, it is vital that you eat right yourself. Spend some time evaluating your own food habits and deciding which ones you want your child to acquire. A parent who is always dieting or skimping on meals day after day will surely have trouble persuading a child to eat well. At the opposite extreme, a parent who is addicted to candy bars, doughnuts, and other junk foods is not in a strong position to lecture a child about choosing foods for their nutritional value and snacking wisely.

You will influence your child's food preferences not only by your own eating, but in other ways as well. Familiarity plays a big part in children's food choices; your child's taste will be strongly influenced and conditioned by the items you serve most often, as well as by what you order when you take her out to a restaurant.

Watching the balance One of the easiest ways to get your child eating healthfully is to serve nutritious foods at every meal. Be sure to offer items from the four basic food groups daily — fruits and vegetables; meats, poultry, and fish; milk and dairy products; and breads and cereals. But do not worry if his diet is not ideally balanced at each meal or even every day. As long as you are providing good food, everything will take care of itself in the end.

However, if you feel you have reason to be concerned, keep track of everything he consumes for a week or two. Write down what he eats (and how much of it) at each meal, and all of his snacks. If reading over this record fails to dispel your worries about your child's diet, discuss the list with his pediatrician.

Getting to know foods of many kinds

To ensure that he will grow up enjoying a wide range of nutritious foods, see that your child encounters many different ones early in his life. Be aware, however, that he may not accept new foods right away — indeed, he may be suspicious of them. This cautious reaction, seen in the young of many species, increases as children grow older and gain more control over their eating. You will probably need to offer a different food repeatedly, so that your youngster has time to become accustomed to it and accept it.

When introducing a new item, it is best to serve a very small portion. Encourage your child to sample a little of it but do not insist. Many children like to investigate the food by simply looking at it, touching it, or smelling it. If your little one does the same, she is not rejecting what you have set before her or deciding never to eat it; she is merely exploring something unknown. Put yourself in her tiny shoes; remember that to a baby, all foods are new.

Keep serving the item in small, introductory portions, giving your child time to get used to it. Let her see you eating the food and let her make her own decision about whether she wants to add it to her diet. But do not be upset if there are foods that she never warms up to, even though you love them. Children, like adults, are entitled to their

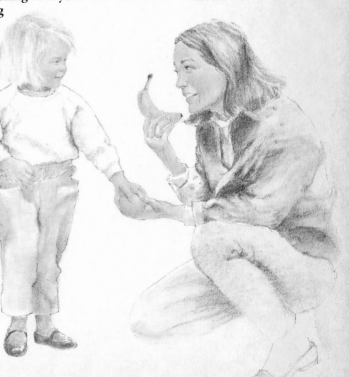

Given a choice between an orange and a banana, a little girl selects the fruit she wants. You can boost your child's interest in her diet by allowing her to make some simple choices about what she eats.

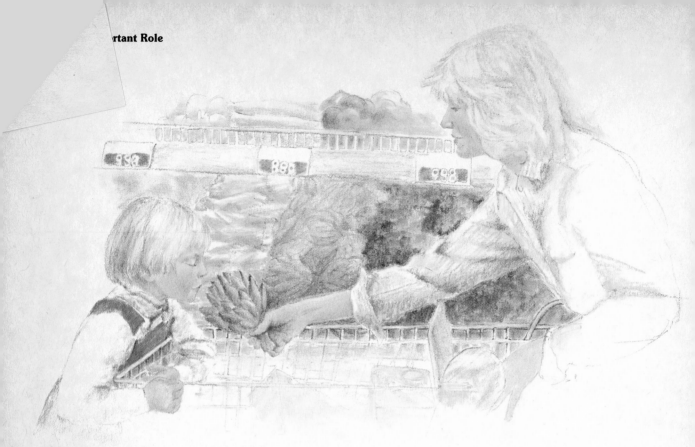

Investigating an item new to him, a boy noses up to an artichoke. Including children in supermarket shopping can make them feel important and arouse their interest in different foods.

personal idiosyncracies, and some want little variety in their diets. Although eating the same foods again and again may seem humdrum to you, an unvaried diet need not be harmful to your youngster's health. She can be just as well nourished by a few familiar favorites, provided that these offer proper balance, as by a spectrum of meats, vegetables, and fruits.

The value of choice

To let your child feel that he has some control over what he eats, offer him choices, being sure that both options are nutritious. A child who is allowed to choose part of his daily menu is more likely to be cooperative about eating the meals you serve him. Be sure to keep in mind his limited decision-making ability and always keep the choices simple. It is better to ask, "Do you want apple juice or milk?" rather than, "What would you like to drink?"

Taking food binges in stride

Children often go on food jags, requesting the same item day after day, then suddenly dropping that food for a new favorite. Such picky eating can try any parent's patience. You cannot prevent these little binges, but you can learn to deal with them in a positive way, comforting yourself with the knowledge that children outgrow them. Often you can decide to play along with the fad of the moment; as long as it fits into a balanced diet, there can be no harm in serving the same favorite lunch or snack for days on end.

Do not, however, let a child's fussy preferences disrupt

family meals. If he will not eat what you have made for the whole family, it is a mistake to let him sweet-talk you into coming up with a separate dish prepared especially for him. Let him pick at a few vegetables and eat a slice of bread; he will most likely recoup his calorie and nutrient losses at the next mealtime or snacktime.

New-food strategies When you are trying to introduce new foods, notice how your child's attitude varies through the day. There may be times when he is hungrier than others and thus more willing to experiment. Offer new items at different mealtimes and snack-times to find out when they get the best reception.

Your child may be invited to eat at the homes of friends, and this can help you widen her food horizons. Talk with her about what she ate at her friend's house and what she especially liked about it. You may get fresh ideas, and you might trade recipes and feeding tips with other children's parents, enriching two households at once.

Let your child assist You can further increase your child's interest in foods and taste experiments by including her in shopping and meal prepara-tion. Share the job of making up your shopping list; let her help you load groceries into your shopping cart, unload them at the check-out counter, and unpack them at home. Later, give her a few simple table-setting tasks. These activities will make her feel involved and boost her excitement over everything about family mealtimes, including the foods you give her to eat.

Naturally, many kitchen chores are dangerous for a young child, especially the ones involving a hot stove. But your child may enjoy even make-believe jobs that resemble your work. For example, dress her in an apron and give her a wooden spoon and a bowl of raw beans or rice to stir, while you are nearby beating a cake batter. Play-cooking will help her feel more at home with the real cooking you are doing and more excited about the food you later put on her plate.

Helping your child eat with ease You can increase your youngster's enthusiasm for her meals by serving food that she can eat easily. You can help your little one eat salads by serving her portion as finger food, without the dressing. Be sure to cut meat into bite-size pieces before serving it to a small child. This saves her the chore of trying— and possible frustration of failing — to cut it herself. And if the meat happens to be on the dry side, always accompany it with moist, creamy, or pureed vegetables.

The Ins and Outs of Shopping with Your Child
- Never leave for the supermarket when you or your youngster is hungry and likely to succumb to impulse buys.
- Give him clear rules for the trip: no running around the store, no candy from the machines, no items that are not on your shopping list.
- Bring a snack such as grapes or crackers for him to munch on while you shop and a small toy for him to play with. You might want to tie the toy to the shopping cart so that you will not have to retrieve it repeat-edly from the floor.
- Put an infant's seat in the shopping cart. If the child can sit up in the cart, use a safety strap.
- Stimulate your youngster's mind as you shop. Talk about weights and measures, where different groceries come from, how empty food containers can be turned into toys.
- Let your youngster select some items from the shelves, place them in the shopping cart, and help unload them at the check-out counter.

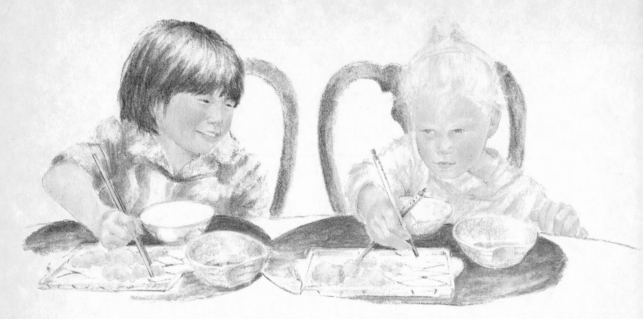

With concentration, a preschooler wields her chopsticks to taste Asian foods at the home of her Japanese-American friend. Youngsters are more likely to try new foods after seeing friends eating them.

Some meats, especially if they are well-done, may be too tough and fibrous for your child to chew, no matter how small the pieces. When you are serving a roast or steak for the family dinner, you may want to give your toddler a hamburger instead. You can keep a few patties of lean ground beef or lamb in the freezer and cook them up as needed. But be careful to cook them slowly, at medium heat, leaving the meat juicy so your child can chew it with ease and pleasure.

Your youngster may enjoy food more if it is served at room temperature: Small children are quite sensitive to heat and cold. By spooning her portion into her dish a few minutes before the meal begins, you can let it warm up or cool down before she touches it. When you make mealtimes easier for your child, you help her to eat with better appetite the dishes you prepare for her.

Making food look good enough to eat

Another way to promote hearty eating is to make sure the food you serve tastes and looks good. This does not mean using herbs or spices or decorating and shaping every item to look like a toy. It does mean realizing that your child will be drawn to food that is carefully cooked and well presented. A sprig of parsley or basil can dress up such plain food as mashed potatoes. A pretty or amusing table setting can further spark your child's appetite. You can add color by using place mats and inexpensive, nonbreakable plastic plates and bowls . Flowers on the table, or candles for special occasions, will enhance the mealtime mood, giving you, your young one, and the rest of the family added pleasure in breaking bread together.

Providing you have the time, you can add interest to your

child's meal by cutting some of the items into interesting shapes. If he will not eat carrot slices, for example, try serving carrot sticks instead or use a wavy blade to produce rippled slices. If your child turns up his nose at a sandwich cut down the middle, try cutting it diagonally or serve it in quarters instead of halves. Tinkering with a food's shape may give a dramatic lift to your child's mealtime enthusiasm.

Giving your child alternatives

Sometimes you may feel that nothing you can do will stimulate your child's interest in a food, in which case remember back to your own childhood preferences and try to be sympathetic. There must have been some items — Brussels sprouts, spinach, liver?—that you persisted in hating, no matter how many chances you had to get used to them. If your child develops a few similar food aversions, try to respect his feelings. His likes and dislikes are now forming and are a valid part of who he is.

Besides, no single food is ever indispensable to health and well-being; among those your child likes, you will always be able to find one that gives him the same nutrients as a food that he hates. A child may flatly reject a cooked vegetable but happily eat the same vegetable raw. Or he may refuse milk but gobble down yogurt or cheese. It does not take much effort to get to know your youngster's food preferences and build a sound diet around them.

Avoid bribery and threats

Guard against the temptation to coax and bribe a child to eat. One of the worst ways you can influence your young one's eating habits is by saying things like, "Eat all your peas or you'll get no dessert," or, "If you clean your plate, you may watch TV after dinner." These feeding tactics may pay off in the short term, but studies show that over time, children learn to dislike the foods they have been badgered into eating. In one study, children had to drink a certain fruit juice before they were allowed to play. At the end of the study, 75 percent of the youngsters liked that juice less than they had at the start. How much better it is to let your child pass up a food she really does not want than to wheedle a few mouthfuls into her and turn her against that food for life.

Bribing children with one food to get them to eat another is especially counterproductive. Parents who use this practice usually offer a sweet dessert as an inducement to eat some unpopular meat or vegetable. Their children simply come to hate the food they are pressured to eat and crave the payoff. In other words, parents who seek to promote good nutritional

Common Concerns

Those Nagging Thoughts

My children want me to be a short-order cook.

Gently but firmly make it clear that your home is not a restaurant where everyone can order a separate meal. If your youngster refuses to touch the main course, let her do with bread, milk, a few bites of salad, and so on. She won't starve.

Should I worry if my child does not want to drink milk?

Drinking milk is a convenient way for your child to get needed nutrients, but it is not essential after infancy. If he doesn't like milk, there is no reason not to substitute other dairy products such as cheese, yogurt, and pudding.

Does my youngster have to eat a good breakfast?

Without a nutritious start to the day, a child's energy will begin to flag by midmorning. Many children, however, are simply not hungry within an hour or so of waking up. For a child who doesn't want to eat before leaving for her day-care center, try packing a cheese sandwich or other nontraditional breakfast for her to eat on the bus or when she gets there. Or you can beat an egg into a glass of milk or juice and serve that for breakfast. Children are often more ready to drink in the morning than they are to eat.

Are junk foods just empty calories?

It depends on what junk foods you're talking about. Ice cream may be full of

sugar, artificial colors, and artificial flavors, but it also offers the nutritional benefits of milk. It can be given as an occasional treat. Even foods with minimal nutrients may be all right for a young child who burns up lots of calories in vigorous play. Snacks can be harmful if they are loaded with fat, salt, and preservatives and fill a child up so that he doesn't eat the fruits, vegetables, and other foods he needs for a balanced diet. Total abstinence from junk food is not necessary, but moderation is essential.

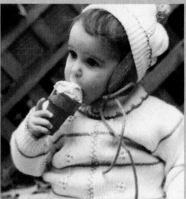

Should I force my child to eat everything that is put before her?

Force-feeding is never a good idea. Children should eat in response to their appetites, not in response to parental pressure. You can avoid many mealtime problems by serving your child small portions and by really meaning it when you urge her, "Try just one bite to see if you like it."

Our kids always finish their meal first and then want their dessert while we're

still eating our dinner. Should we serve it to them right away?

You don't want to punish your children for finishing before you by making them endure a boring, fidgety period of inactivity while you eat the rest of your meal. Nor do you want them to regard dessert as a reward they get for sitting around watching you eat. If you approve of the dessert as part of your children's diet, go ahead and give it to them when they're ready for it.

Should I take my child's dinner away when he doesn't eat and tell him he won't get anything until morning?

Refusing to eat at the times you set, like refusing the food you serve, can be a child's way of making a bid for autonomy. If your child is testing the limits of your control in this way, it's fine to be firm about family mealtimes and to make it clear that passing up dinner will mean going hungry until breakfast. Your youngster won't waste away as a result of going without food for a few hours.

Do children know what kind of food is good for them?

No. Ever since a study done in the 1920s, in which children were allowed to pick what they wanted to eat and selected a healthful diet for themselves, people have believed that youngsters are capable of taking care of their own nutritional needs instinctively. But that study included no sweet foods. A more recent study has shown that when the choice was between a healthful item and a sweet one, the children invariably picked the food containing sugar.

habits by using this method will only defeat their own purpose.

Try never to use food as a reward. Good eating and good discipline (including good table manners) are important, but they are separate issues and should stay separate. You want your child to eat because he is hungry and because he likes the food in front of him, not because the food has become a prize. At times when you feel you must present a food in a reward context, as after a particularly important behavioral achievement, give him something nourishing accompanied by love, praise, and hugs. Teaching him to associate these good feelings with his achievement helps him toward a lifetime of self-motivated good eating.

Watch out for television

No matter how much nutritional guidance your child receives from you, she will be subjected to powerful influences that tend to undermine good eating principles. Not least of these is television. The average American child sees more than 20,000 commercials each year, more than half of them for food products. Cereals, especially sugared cereals, are the items most often pitched to young viewers, followed by snack foods, soft drinks, and flavored vitamins. A child who eats a balanced diet does not need vitamin pills shaped like TV characters, and the other food products advertised on children's programs are of questionable nutritional value at best. Those items that contain large amounts of sugar put the youngsters who eat them at risk for obesity and tooth decay.

The ads promoting these foods are expensive, flashy, and made to be particularly attractive to children. Scientific research has confirmed what parents already knew — that television food ads strongly influence children's eating preferences. They are a factor you must cope with as you guide your youngster's eating habits and nutritional growth.

You can minimize the influence of these ads by watching some of your child's shows with her, and discussing the programs and the ads. Limit her commercial television time by providing other diversions, including perhaps a half hour spent viewing an educational show on public television, or reading a good book together. Perhaps most important, you can be firm about refusing to be swayed by any ads for unhealthful food products and say a loving but firm no to your child's inevitable begging. It is not always easy to raise a healthy eater amid television's pervasive antinutrition messages, but it is possible, and the benefits to your child's health and growth are certainly well worth the effort. ∴

A Guide to Equipment

Simple though it may be, the basic equipment a child uses at mealtime — bottles, bibs, cups, dishes, utensils, high chair — can have strong bearing on how she behaves and how well she eats. A thoughtfully designed piece can actually speed the process by which a youngster learns to feed herself. An awkward one — a nipple that clogs, a clumsy spoon, an uncomfortable high chair — can frustrate offspring and parent alike. In addition, a well-designed item can minimize mess, eliminating unnecessary cleanup work.

Here, for your guidance, is a range of commonly available equipment, from everyday necessities to optional extras, with pointers on practicality and safety.

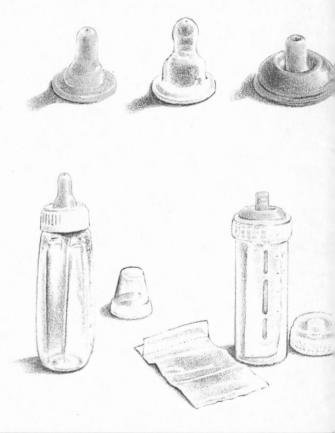

Nipples

Your baby is bound to take to some nipples and hate others, which makes choosing the right one a trial-and-error process. Instead of buying a dozen nipples right off, try one out on your child first. Consider the following:

● Nipples are available with various hole diameters, each for a different liquid: a small hole for water, a larger one for thicker liquids such as orange juice. The hole should allow a steady, slow trickle of fluid when you invert the bottle. Too small a hole frustrates the baby and clogs easily; if the hole is too large, the baby may choke on fast-flowing fluids. Never use so-called cross-cut nipples, which have extra-large holes designed for diluted cereals; not only can a young baby choke on the flow, but they get in the way of the child's own innate ability to regulate his caloric intake.

● Nipples are available in various sizes and shapes, and the type you choose should be largely a matter of your baby's preference. The nipple's tip should rest against the palate near the front of the baby's mouth; a nipple that is too long or too large is hard for the baby to control. Round nipples (*near right*) are the most familiar, having been around for years. Many pediatricians recommend so-called orthodontic nipples (*center*), which conform to the palate, but these can be too large for premature or small infants. The nipples for widely available disposable bottles are made extra-broad to fit the bottles' wide mouths (*far right*).

● Nipples are made of two materials. The most durable is silicone (*center*), a material that holds up through many sterilizations and does not stain. The more traditional latex rubber nipple is as functional but has a shorter lifespan. Latex nipples (*near and far right*) should be discarded when they discolor, become sticky, peel, or crack.

Bottles

Standard bottles (*near right*), complete with nipple, screw-on plastic collar, and cover are available in various materials. Glass, ideal for feeding the newborn, is scratchproof, easy to clean and sterilize, but breakable. Clear, rigid plastic, better for toddlers, is light enough for a young child to hold and is virtually indestructible, although it scratches easily and can stain. Flexible, opaque plastic bottles and those with odd shapes absorb stains and are hard to clean. An alternative to the bottle is a disposable nursing system (*opposite, bottom right*), with a special nipple and cover, a screw-on collar, a bottle-shaped plastic holder, and a sterile, throwaway plastic bag for the liquid. Such nursers need no sterilizing, but they have some disadvantages: Fluids cannot be accurately measured or diluted, the bags sometimes leak, and some babies dislike the unusual nipple shape.

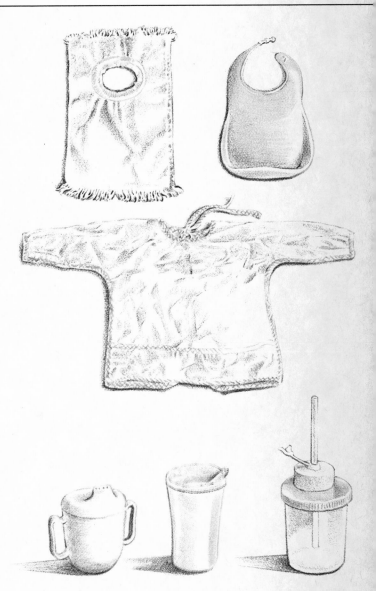

Bibs

Children are such messy eaters that a big bib is essential, although no bib yet invented can keep a determined child from wearing her food. The traditional terry cloth bib, either with a stretch collar that slips over the head (*near right*) or with adjustable ties or fasteners, absorbs spills well but needs frequent laundering. A stiff plastic bib (*far right*) with a catch pocket not only catches spilled or dropped food but can be wiped clean. Some children find the stiffness uncomfortable, however. A plastic, long-sleeved coverall bib (*center*), especially useful for active toddlers, provides the most protection and is easy to clean. But getting a child into and out of it can be a chore, and your youngster may dislike such a constricting and warm garment. Like any piece of flexible plastic, the coverall bib can pose a hazard if an unattended child covers her face with it and is unable to breathe; it should be used only when an adult is present.

Drinking Cups

Cups vary in design and practicality according to the ages of the children for whom they are intended. A baby's first cup (*near right*) needs to be strong, stable, and easy to use. It should be made of thick plastic that cannot be bitten through or smashed when dropped. It should have a wide, weighted base to guard against tipping and a snap cap or screw cap with a drinking spout to prevent spilling and to smooth the transition from bottle to cup. And it should have double handles for easier control. As a child gains skill, he can switch to a taller, straight-sided cup (*center*), with or without a top. Eventually he will want to drink from a straw; the special lid at far right accommodates a straw while keeping the contents from spilling.

Utensils

Learning to use a spoon, knife, and fork is a years-long process that cannot be rushed. When you first introduce solid food to your baby around four to six months, you can use the long-handled spoon shown at near right, which has a rubber-coated bowl to protect gums and teeth. Although she will soon begin playing with the spoon, she will not be ready to shift from feeding herself with her fingers to manipulating a spoon until she is nine to twelve months old.

When she is ready, you can introduce a baby spoon, with a shallow, wide bowl and short, thick handle. A spoon that has a looped handle (*second from left*) is easiest for a novice to hold, while a curved handle (*third from left*) will aid any child who has trouble with the dexterous wrist-bending movement involved in straight-handled spoon use. Once she has the knack of eating with a baby spoon, she can graduate to a sturdy straight-handled spoon like the one shown here (*center*).

When your child is about two and a half years old, she can begin using a child's fork (*third from right*), which has short, blunt tines. If necessary, you can provide a squeegeelike pusher (*second from right*) to help her load food onto a spoon or fork.

At three or four years old, preschoolers learn to use knives (*far right*) as spreaders. Choose a short-handled knife that has a rounded tip and a dull cutting edge. Then, at about the age of five, when your child can butter bread with aplomb, she can start using the same knife to cut up her food — the final step to self-sufficiency at the dinner table.

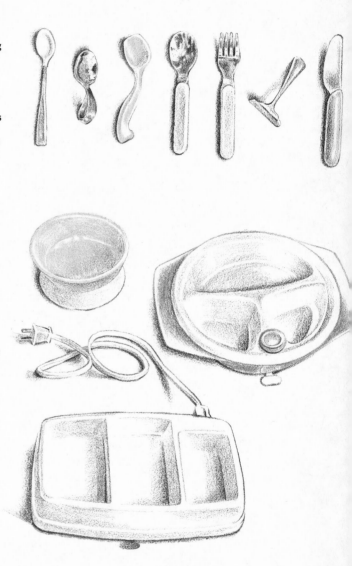

Dishes

Soon after you start spoon-feeding your baby, you will need to introduce him to dishes — first for finger foods, then for his whole diet. The best dish for a toddler is a deep bowl (*center, left*) with steep sides, against which the child can scoop his spoon. A bowl with a suction base is ideal; it will hold steady and prevent spills. Often such a bowl will come with a convenient tab release — preferably one that does not easily yield to an enterprising two-year-old. And the bowl should be made of thick, unbreakable, dishwasher-proof plastic.

Persnickety preschoolers who hate to mix different foods sometimes prefer compartmented dishes. Slow eaters are well served by dishes that keep food warm. These come in two types. The hot-water warmer (*center, right*) has a dish mounted over a compartment that can be easily filled with hot tap water (never boiling water). It should have a large, tightly fitting cap that your child cannot easily remove. This guards against his swallowing the cap or scalding himself. An electric warmer (*bottom*) has a built-in heating coil that permits the dish to be warmed for a few minutes before food is served. The cord then is detached and latent heat keeps the contents warm for a half hour or so.

High Chairs and Drop Cloths

Once your six-month-old can confidently sit by herself, she is ready for a high chair. These come in two types: those that can be folded and those that are rigid. Make sure the base is much wider than the seat, so that the most energetic child cannot tip the chair. In buying a collapsible high chair, look for one that has a securely locking mechanism that will not pinch you or your child. The chair's back should be high enough to support her head and its footrest should be sturdy; chairs in which these are adjustable are more comfortable for the growing child. The seat should be fitted with both an easy-to-use safety belt and a crotch strap to keep the baby from sliding under the tray. The wide, wraparound tray should be removable for cleaning, with secure, convenient latches that will not pinch or scratch you or your baby. And the tray should have a lip to catch spills.

Even with such a tray, food is bound to fall to the floor. The easiest way to avoid a mess is to spread a drop cloth (*top*) under the chair. It can be shaken and wiped clean when the mealtime is over.

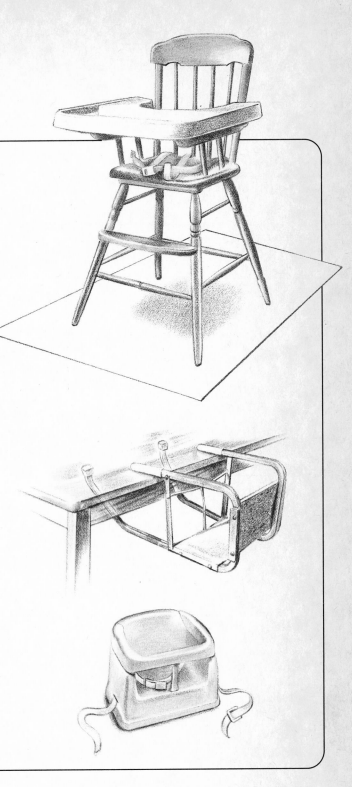

Portable High Chairs

Away from home, a portable, folding high chair (*center*) vastly simplifies meals. Most portable chairs grip a table edge and allow a baby to eat from the table. They should have a secure gripping mechanism and all the important attributes of a regular high chair, especially safety belts, crotch straps, and pinch-proof locking mechanisms.

Booster Seats

When a child outgrows his high chair but is not yet tall enough to reach the table from a dining-room chair, he needs a booster seat. Often made of molded plastic, the best booster seats have a deep seating well, a crotch strap or bar, and safety straps that fasten the seat to a dining-room chair.

Making Mealtimes Work

Although a family meal is a social event, it is not automatically a happy time for a toddler or preschooler. Sitting still for a long time is hard for him, and he may feel left out of adult conversation. Then, too, his behavior at the table may sometimes upset you and provoke responses that you and he will both regret. By knowing the potential problems and preventing them or meeting them positively, you will nurture your child's development and set the stage for a lifetime of eating pleasure and good health.

Transition time before a meal

Help your child come to dinner in the best possible frame of mind. Do not call her directly from play to the table. She may be too tired, or too wound up, to notice that she is hungry. Give her at least a fifteen-minute warning before dinner actually begins so that she has plenty of time to simmer down and wash her hands. Assign her a table-setting task geared to her age; this will help orient her toward eating. When you praise her for her accomplishment, she will be pleased with herself and all the more ready to help the next time she is asked. If you can manage it, spend a few minutes with her in reading or some other quiet activity to help her slow down and prepare herself to enjoy the meal.

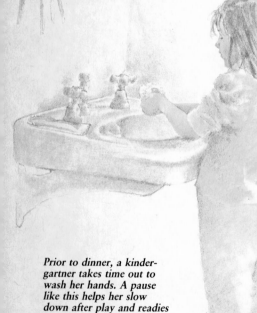

Prior to dinner, a kindergartner takes time out to wash her hands. A pause like this helps her slow down after play and readies her for the period when she will have to sit still.

When everyone is seated at the table, be prepared to let your child have as much time to eat as he needs. Small children often eat slowly and will not do their best if they feel they are being rushed through a meal. And again, remember that your child's stomach is smaller than yours. He may eat his fill before you are finished, then want to get down and play, especially if sitting at the table with the rest of the family is something he has not done before. Forcing him to sit with you after he is done will be pleasant for no one, so let him go. He may return for the odd bite before the meal is over. When he has had more dinner-table experience, you can introduce a rule: Leaving the table means that for him, the meal is over.

Make an effort to keep the atmosphere cheerful and comfortable during the meal.

Do not use this family time to argue or give vent to grievances. And more important, do not scold your youngster or harangue her about the way she is eating. The dinner table should never become a battleground.

One way to ensure relaxed mealtimes is to keep your concerns about your child's diet and nutrition separate from other issues, such as ethical standards and family discipline. You may talk about food, certainly, but however important teaching your child to obey your authority and sharing your moral values with her may be to you, they are all different from the job of nourishing her properly and should not be allowed as part of mealtime. Keep the distinctions clear in your own mind, and you will spare her a great deal of potential conflict and confusion.

No force feedings   Mealtime becomes a miserable clash of wills when parents attempt to force a child to eat, purely as a way of teaching her to do what she is told. You want to train your youngster to be aware of her appetite, to feed herself a wholesome diet, and to know when she is hungry and when she is full. These goals will

Delighting in one another's company, three friends share a snack at their own child-size table. Researchers have found what parents already knew: Children will sit longer and eat more in the company of their peers.

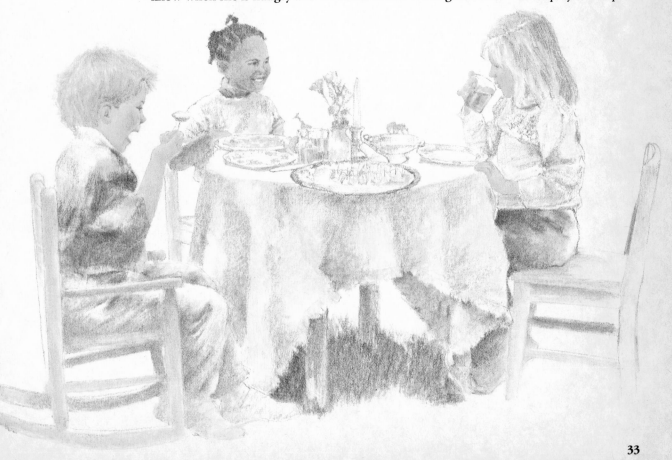

suffer if you insist on playing the tyrant at mealtime, substituting your demands for her natural self-feeding instincts. Furthermore, your heavy-handed approach will only encourage your youngster to dig in her heels and become stubborn just to defy you. If you do not force her to eat in order to prove your authority, your child will not need to use rejection of food as a way of asserting her autonomy.

A relaxed approach to table manners

Just as you may feel impelled to discipline your child about his eating, you may be tempted to take angry or punitive measures to control his table manners. It can be hard to endure a very young child's wild, messy mealtime behavior, but a gentle, patient approach to this matter works far better than impatient shouts, threats, or punishments. Remember first of all that table manners are a separate issue from eating. A child who is by adult standards a careless and impolite table companion may nevertheless still be feeding himself a healthful diet. Keep in mind, too, that the friendly mealtime atmosphere that promotes good eating is also the best setting for helping a youngster acquire proper table manners.

To teach your child how to behave at the table, start with the simplest basics. A three-year-old can deal with the rudiments of neat eating and politeness, but he should not be expected to grasp the finer points of mealtime etiquette. Go easy on him and be tolerant of his lapses. Accept that undesirable behavior will change slowly, and that progress will be accompanied by some backsliding. Do not bombard your child with orders and reprimands; coach him gently instead. He will learn slowly, but in the end he will learn.

You can start to practice firm but gentle mealtime discipline when your child is still eating in a baby table or high chair. Babies often take great interest in playing with their food — rubbing it on their faces, or smearing and doodling in it with their fingers. Allow a bit of this activity; it is your infant's way of exploring her food and enjoying its smell and texture. But have firm guidelines about when to call a halt and take the meal away. Generally, you should remove food when your baby starts to throw it, especially those new items you are trying out on her. Do not react to food throwing and other common infant behaviors in any way that would encourage her to do it again. For example, when your baby grimaces and spits a gob of strained carrots down her chin, suppress your laugh unless you want her to think that this act pleases you and should be repeated just to keep you entertained.

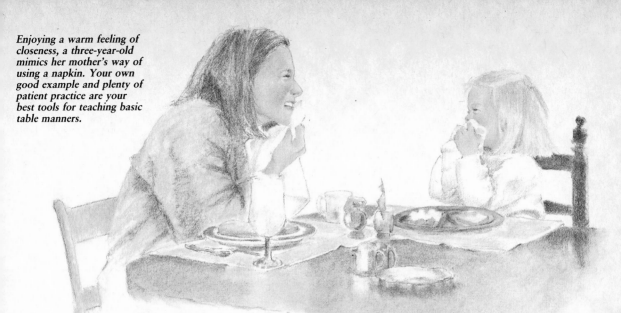

Enjoying a warm feeling of closeness, a three-year-old mimics her mother's way of using a napkin. Your own good example and plenty of patient practice are your best tools for teaching basic table manners.

When your child begins to play with his food

An older child does not play with food as extravagantly as a baby does, but there often comes a point in a meal when he stops eating it and begins fooling around with it. The best response is simply to remove his plate, with no negative comment. You are not punishing him; you are simply recognizing that he has finished eating. Use the same approach when he grows restless and fidgety and starts playing at the table. Instead of scolding him and forcing him to sit still, let him excuse himself.

Offering an example and positive reinforcement

Remember that your child learns most of her table manners by watching you. Since your example is her main influence, the best way to ensure that she says "please" and "thank you" is always to use those magic words yourself. After personal example, the most effective teaching method is reinforcing desirable behavior. Make a point of praising your youngster when she is eating nicely. Respond to misbehavior, especially when it is disrupting the family meal, by simply removing her without comment from the table.

The need for physical comfort

Your child's physical comfort when eating contributes much to his mealtime happiness and good behavior. Seat him so that his food is within easy reach at belly level, and his feet have something to rest on and do not dangle. Give him dishes and utensils that he can use easily to feed himself. You can buy special child-size silverware or simply give him a small, broad salad fork. Serve his food on a small plate, deep enough that he can use the rim for help in scooping food onto his fork or spoon. For minimum spilling, let him drink from a glass with a broad base. Since some food is bound to fall to the floor beneath his seat, you may want to protect the floor with a drop cloth. Physical arrangements such as these create a positive emotional atmosphere and help make family meals pleasant learning experiences for your child. ❖

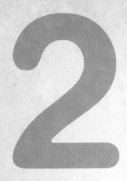

A World of Choice

The little girl savoring a crisp, juicy apple at right has acquired a taste for healthful food that will sustain her for a lifetime. But her love for apples did not simply happen; children do not come into the world with predetermined food preferences. Rather, they develop their eating habits slowly, learning from what they are fed in the early years of life.

As a loving parent, you naturally want to provide your child with all the nutrients and calories she needs to grow and develop. But how? Food fads and seemingly contradictory information on television and in the newspapers and magazines can confuse the issue. A good place to start is here with the facts about nutrition presented in this section. Armed with basic information, you can make wise food purchases at the supermarket and plan wholesome menus that will meet your child's needs for protein, carbohydrates, fats, minerals, and vitamins. Knowing which foods contain which nutrients is the first step toward providing a well-balanced diet.

Remember too that your youngster's nutritional requirements are different from your own. Because you eat well, it does not necessarily follow that she will if you give her the same foods you like. Besides the nutrients necessary to maintain her present size, she needs additional nutrients to build the tissue that is forever multiplying in her body and to supply the energy she burns off living and learning.

Fortunately, nutrition is not an arcane science. Healthy eating is largely a matter of common sense with diversity and moderation the watchwords. If your child learns to eat a variety of foods at a young age, chances are excellent that she will continue to enjoy a healthful, diversified diet for the rest of her life.

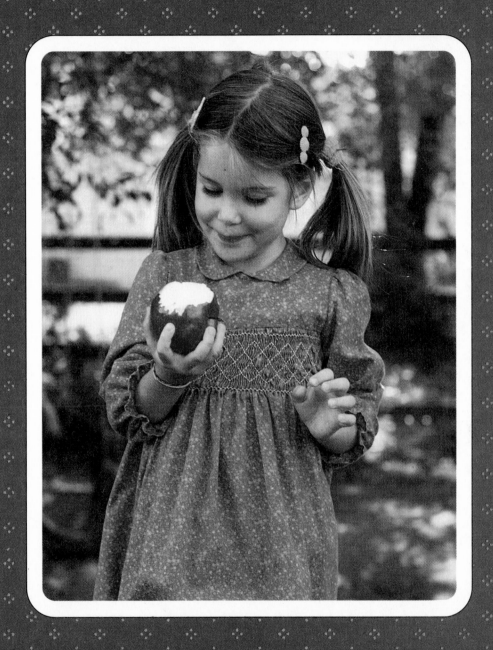

Nutrients: The Body's Building Blocks

Simply put, nutrition is the way the body takes in and uses food. The process works like this: The digestive system breaks the food down into nutrients — chemical substances that promote growth, build and maintain cells, and help regulate body processes. The nutrients are then absorbed by the intestines and acted upon by metabolic processes within the liver and other organs. Finally the substances are absorbed into tissues, to be stored for future use or burned for energy.

Types of nutrients

Children, like adults, need at least fifty different types of nutrients. These can be divided into six categories — proteins, carbohydrates, fats, vitamins, minerals, and water. Carbohydrates, proteins, and fats are macronutrients, so called because the body needs fairly large quantities of them. They make up the bulk of your child's daily nutrient intake. Vitamins and minerals are known as micronutrients since they are present in food in much smaller quantities. Scientists measure them in milligrams and micrograms. If you want to know how infinitesimally small these amounts are, think of an ordinary paper clip as weighing about a gram; a milligram is one-thousandth of a gram and a microgram is one-thousandth of a milligram.

Among the fifty macro- and micronutrients, ten — protein, carbohydrates, fat, vitamins A, C, B_1, B_2, B_3, calcium, and iron — are referred to as leader nutrients. If your child has a balanced diet, she will receive all ten in the amounts she requires. And a balanced diet will almost certainly contain the other forty nutrients as well. In addition, remember that essential nutrient, water. She must obtain it in sufficient quantities to ensure that nutrients are carried to her cells and waste products swept away.

Since no single food contains all the leader nutrients, it is important that your growing child consume a variety of foods. Concentrating on meat or potatoes or bread, no matter how nutritious each may be, is no substitute for eating a balanced diet; an extra supply of one nutrient in the body cannot compensate for the shortage of another. A child who is undernourished over a long period will be irritable, inattentive, and apathetic. Worse, if the condition persists, her growth and development will be delayed, even stunted, and resistance to disease lowered. ❖

Starting at the grass-roots level, a robust toddler digs in a vegetable patch. Six months earlier he was still a baby; a healthy diet has helped him grow strong.

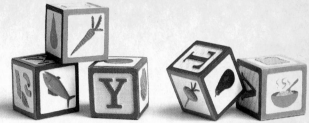

Fulfilling Your Youngster's Basic Nutritional Needs

Daily Allowances

Nutrition is a science, with nutritionists working to exacting standards to determine the energy needs that food must supply and the amount of each nutrient the average healthy child or adult should have in his diet. Energy needs are measured in heat units called calories. Nutritional requirements are expressed by the U.S. National Academy of Sciences as the Recommended Dietary Allowances, or RDAs, that you see on nutrition labels. Neither the caloric nor the RDA recommendations, however, should be considered rigid daily formulas. In fact, the experts who devised them suggest that people average out their consumption of nutrients over a five- to eight-day period. Thus you do not have to be overly concerned if your child's diet lacks a particular nutrient for a few days, so long as over the course of a week or two, she gets food containing that nutrient in an amount sufficient to fulfill her need. For help in translating the RDAs on the chart that follows into practical food applications, see the food guide on page 50. It gives the number of suggested servings per day from the four basic food groups and portion sizes appropriate for toddlers and preschoolers.

Caloric Requirements

The fuel that keeps your active child going comes from the calories she consumes. Calories are derived from three basic groups of nutrients — fats, carbohydrates, and proteins. They enable your youngster's muscles, brain, and nerves to function and are essential for the production of tissue. All children require more calories per pound of body weight than adults need. A child who receives too few calories will grow at a less than normal rate. Remember that each child is unique; your youngster's rate of development and sense of well-being should be your final yardstick in determining her energy needs.

Daily Recommendations
Birth to 12 months: 40 to 60 calories per pound per day
1 to 3 years: 35 to 45 calories per pound per day
4 to 6 years: 20 to 35 calories per pound per day
Sources
All foods.

Water

Water is essential to life; it is a nutrient that performs many important tasks. In addition to dissolving and carrying other nutrients and wastes to and from cells within the body, it helps to regulate body temperature and to lubricate the system.

The water requirements of children are greater than those of adults. Indeed, the water content of an infant is about ten percent higher than that of a grown-up. Babies need ten to fifteen percent of their lean body weight a day in fluids, while older children must have three ounces of fluids for every 100 calories they burn.

Fortunately, the natural food of infants — breast milk — is high in water, as is formula. Keep in mind that a child's body, like an adult's, responds to built-in thirst signals; your youngster will let you know when he is thirsty.

Daily Recommendations
Birth to 6 months: 2.3 to 1.7 ounces per pound
6 to 12 months: 1.7 ounces per pound
1 to 3 years: 1.7 to 1.0 ounces per pound
4 to 6 years: 1.0 ounces per pound
Sources
Liquids and all foods, except dried ones.

Protein

Throughout a lifetime, the body needs protein to maintain and repair cell tissue; to make hemoglobin which carries oxygen to the cells; to build antibodies for combating disease and infection; and to produce hormones and enzymes that regulate body processes. In infancy and childhood, protein is necessary for growth. Children use theirs quickly; unlike some nutrients, it cannot be stored in the body, which means that supplies must be replenished daily. In general, 10 to 15 percent of a child's daily calories should come from protein.

There are two types of protein: complete and incomplete. Complete proteins contain enough of the essential amino acids or building blocks that the body needs for normal metabolism. They occur mostly in foods of animal origin. Incomplete proteins are found in such plant products as peas, beans, nuts, seeds, grains, and tofu. They are called incomplete because they contain far fewer essential amino acids, and must be eaten in combination with one another to be fully useful to the body (*page 55*).

Daily Recommendations
These figures are for children leading normal lives, full of active play.
Birth to 6 months: 1 gram per pound of body weight
6 to 12 months: .9 grams per pound
1 to 3 years: .8 grams per pound
4 to 6 years: .7 grams per pound
Sources
Meat, poultry, fish, eggs, milk, legumes, nuts.

Carbohydrates

Carbohydrates, which provide the body's immediate source of energy, fall into two groups. Complex carbohydrates are the starches found in rice, some vegetables such as corn and potatoes, and bread and cereals; these are broken down by the body to provide glucose, its fuel. Simple carbohydrates are the readily absorbed sugars — which require less breaking down — present in vegetables and fruit. Both should be plentiful in a child's diet, so that her body can use protein for growth.

Daily Recommendations

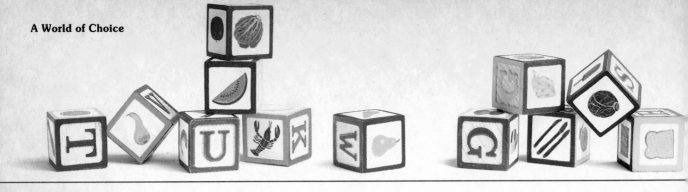

Birth to 6 years: 25 to 55 percent of all calories
Sources
Whole grains, legumes, potatoes, corn, fruits, nuts, milk.

Fats

As an essential part of a growing child's diet, fat provides, ounce for ounce, more energy when it is oxidized or burned by the body than any other nutrient. But it does a great deal more. Liquid fat carries vitamins A, D, E, and K, which cannot dissolve in water, to the cells. As your child's only source of linoleic acid, fat promotes normal growth and healthy skin. In its stored form, it cushions such vital organs as the kidneys and acts as insulation, protecting the body from excessive heat loss.

Actually, there are three different kinds of fat: saturated, polyunsaturated, and monounsaturated. Saturated fat occurs in foods of animal origin; the greater the saturation or density of the fat itself, the harder it will be at room temperature, which is why butter, consisting of 59 percent saturated fat, firms up when chilled. Saturated fat tends to raise blood levels of cholesterol, a fatty substance manufactured by the body and present in all animal fat. As deposits of cholesterol build up in the arteries, they increase the risk of heart disease by constricting the flow of blood to the heart. By contrast, polyunsaturated fat, produced by plants, maintains and even lowers blood levels of cholesterol; it exists in abundance in safflower and other vegetable oils. Monounsaturated fat, also produced by plants and a big component of olive and peanut oils, may play a similarly useful role in the regulation of blood cholesterol levels.

However vital it is to human existence, fat is still a nutrient to watch. When consumed to excess, it leads, of course, to unnecessary weight gain, and there is the danger of cholesterol buildup. For these reasons, parents should encourage their children over the age of two to eat a diet that provides no more than 35 percent of its calories from fat (*page 53*). This is especially true if your family has a history of heart disease. A word of warning, however: Children under the age of two should not be given a low-fat diet; it may severely limit their caloric intake, which in turn may stop or retard normal growth and development.

Daily Recommendations
Birth to 2 years: 50 percent of all calories
2 to 6 years: 30 to 35 percent of all calories
Sources
Meat, fish, dairy products, vegetable oils, margarine, milk.

Vitamins

Occurring in all foods, vitamins are organic compounds essential for normal body functions and growth: While they are not sources of energy, they are necessary for the transformation of protein, carbohydrates, and fat into energy.

The thirteen vitamins needed by humans are absorbed into the body two ways. Four — A, D, E, and K — are fat-soluble; that is, they must dissolve in fat to be absorbed. Since they can be held in reserve in body fat, they do not have to be eaten daily. The water-soluble vitamins — vitamin C and the eight B vitamins — are absorbed and utilized with the aid of water and remain in tissues in small quantities. Any excess amount, however, is excreted in urine. Still, water-soluble vitamins, like the fat-soluble ones, need not be replenished daily, so long as they are part of the weekly diet.

Although vitamin deficiencies can lead to serious health problems, there is little reason for alarm among parents who are feeding their children a well-rounded diet. Youngsters who eat three meals and two nutritious snacks a day that include items from the four basic food groups (*page 50*) get all the vitamins they need. They should not be given vitamin supplements unless these are specifically called for by a doctor: Overdoses of some vitamins can be harmful. Too much vitamin A, for example, can cause a host of physical problems, ranging from blurred vision and loss of appetite to liver damage and abnormal bone growth. Bear in mind, however, that it is almost impossible for your child to receive too much of a particular vitamin through food alone.

Vitamin A. Fat-Soluble

Essential for bone growth, vitamin A is also needed for night and color vision and healthy skin. It enables the body to repair its cells, especially the mucous membranes of the eyelids, eyes, nose, mouth, and digestive tract.

Daily Recommendations
The RDAs for vitamin A traditionally include the notation RE, which stands for retinol equivalents, the amount of retinol, or active vitamin A, that a vitamin A compound will yield after conversion in the body.
Birth to 6 months: 420 micrograms RE
6 months to 3 years: 400 micrograms RE
4 to 6 years: 500 micrograms RE
Sources
Liver, dairy products, yellow-orange fruits and vegetables, green leafy vegetables, egg yolk.

Vitamin B₁ (Thiamin). Water-Soluble

This vitamin helps break down carbohydrates for energy, promotes a good appetite, and keeps the central nervous system functioning properly.
Daily Recommendations
Birth to 6 months: 0.3 milligrams
6 to 12 months: 0.5 milligrams
1 to 3 years: 0.7 milligrams
4 to 6 years: 0.9 milligrams
Sources
Lean meat, fish, shellfish, whole-grain and enriched cereals and breads, nuts and seeds, legumes, dairy products.

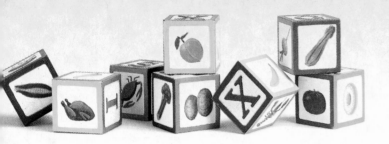
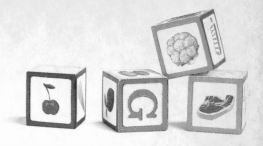

Vitamin B$_2$ (Riboflavin). Water-Soluble

Vitamin B$_2$ helps convert carbohydrates into energy and promotes healthy skin and good vision in bright light.

Daily Recommendations
Birth to 6 months: 0.4 milligrams
6 to 12 months: 0.6 milligrams
1 to 3 years: 0.8 milligrams
4 to 6 years: 1.0 milligrams

Sources
Whole-grain and enriched cereals and breads, dairy products, eggs, meat, liver and other organs, fish, legumes, leafy greens.

Vitamin B$_3$ (Niacin). Water-Soluble

Working in conjunction with vitamins B$_1$ and B$_2$, vitamin B$_3$ aids the body in producing energy from carbohydrates. It also contributes to healthy skin and nerves. Because B$_3$ dissolves easily in water, foods rich in it should be cooked in a minimum of water and the cooking liquid should be used, whenever possible, in sauces or in soups and stews to conserve that portion of the nutrient that dissolved into the liquid.

Daily Recommendations
Birth to 6 months: 6 milligrams
6 to 12 months: 8 milligrams
1 to 3 years: 9 milligrams
4 to 6 years: 11 milligrams

Sources
Meat, poultry, fish, eggs, whole-grain or enriched cereals and breads, nuts, potatoes, tomatoes, mushrooms, legumes, dark green vegetables.

Vitamin B$_6$ (Pyridoxine). Water-Soluble

This B vitamin is needed for the formation of red blood cells and for the body's absorption of carbohydrates, proteins, and fats. The greater the amount of protein in the diet, the greater is the necessity for this vitamin, which is essential to protein metabolism.

Daily Recommendations
Birth to 6 months: 0.3 milligrams
6 to 12 months: 0.6 milligrams
1 to 3 years: 0.9 milligrams
4 to 6 years: 1.3 milligrams

Sources
Whole-grain (but not refined) cereals and bread, meat, liver and kidney, poultry, fish, green leafy vegetables, bananas, avocados, nuts, potatoes, soybeans.

Vitamin B$_{12}$ (Cobalamin). Water-Soluble

This vitamin is necessary for the building of genetic material, the formation of red blood cells, and a healthy nervous system. Infants breast fed by mothers who eat no animal products and children raised as strict vegetarians, with no eggs or milk in their diet, will develop a B$_{12}$ deficiency unless they are given a supplement. Most cases of vitamin B$_{12}$ deficiency, however, are caused by a rare genetic inability to absorb the nutrient.

Daily Recommendations
Birth to 6 months: 0.5 micrograms
6 to 12 months: 1.5 micrograms
1 to 3 years: 2.0 micrograms
4 to 6 years: 2.5 micrograms

Sources
Meat, dairy products, fish, eggs.

Vitamin C. Water-Soluble

Also known as ascorbic acid, Vitamin C promotes healthy gums, teeth, and bones; helps wounds heal; aids in resisting infection; and enhances the body's absorption of iron. It also helps blood vessels stay elastic and strong, thus leaving the body less vulnerable to bruising. Because vitamin C is easily destroyed when exposed to air, light, and heat, foods high in this vitamin should be eaten raw or cooked quickly, preferably in a small amount of liquid or in a microwave oven.

Daily Recommendations
Birth to 12 months: 35 milligrams
1 to 6 years: 45 milligrams

Sources
Citrus fruits, cabbage, green peppers, tomatoes, potatoes, dark green vegetables.

Vitamin D. Fat-Soluble

Vitamin D makes it possible for the body to absorb the minerals calcium and phosphorus, which are crucial for the formation and maintenance of bones and teeth. Occurring naturally in some foods, Vitamin D is also made by sunlight acting on the skin.

Daily Recommendations
Birth to 6 years: 10 micrograms

Sources
Fortified milk, fortified margarine, egg yolks, liver, tuna, salmon.

Vitamin E. Fat-Soluble

Essential for growth, healthy skin and muscles, and the formation of red blood cells, vitamin E also prevents vitamin A from being destroyed and fat from being burned up too rapidly by the body.

Daily Recommendations
Vitamin E is measured in terms of Alpha tocopherol equivalents, the active form of vitamin E utilized by the body.
Birth to 6 months: 3 milligrams Alpha tocopherol equivalents
6 to 12 months: 4 milligrams Alpha tocopherol equivalents
1 to 3 years: 5 milligrams Alpha tocopherol equivalents
4 to 6 years: 6 milligrams Alpha tocopherol equivalents

Sources
Vegetable oils, margarine, wheat germ, whole-grain breads and

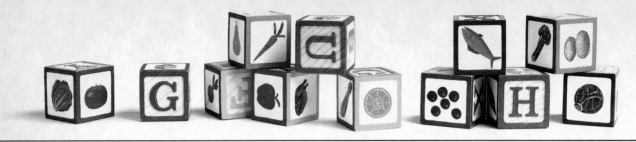

cereals, soybeans, raw or sprouted seeds, sweet potatoes, nuts, liver, green leafy vegetables.

Folic acid (Folacin)

Folic acid works with B_{12} to synthesize genetic material and to form red blood cells. Babies who receive most of their calories from goat's milk, which lacks folic acid and B_{12}, may develop a deficiency, two symptoms of which are diarrhea and anemia, unless given a supplement.

Daily Recommendations
Birth to 6 months: 30 micrograms
6 to 12 months: 45 micrograms
1 to 3 years: 100 micrograms
4 to 6 years: 200 micrograms
Sources
Liver, dark green leafy vegetables, wheat germ, dairy products, legumes.

Vitamin K. Fat-Soluble

Essential for blood clotting and bone development, vitamin K is produced by harmless bacteria acting on foods in the large and small intestines. Most hospitals give newborns an injection of vitamin K soon after birth because the infants' bodies contain so little of it. Intestinal bacteria, breast milk, and fortified formulas provide sufficient vitamin K for older babies.

Daily Recommendations
Birth to 6 months: 12 micrograms
6 to 12 months: 10 to 20 micrograms
1 to 3 years: 15 to 30 micrograms
4 to 6 years: 20 to 40 micrograms
Sources
Green leafy vegetables, cabbage, cauliflower, peas, potatoes, liver, tomatoes, yogurt (the bacteria in yogurt stimulate vitamin K production by the human intestine).

Minerals

Although inorganic, minerals, like vitamins, are crucial to the growth and proper functioning of the body. The minerals needed in relatively large amounts are calcium, phosphorus, magnesium, potassium, sodium, and chloride. Those needed in only small amounts include iron, zinc, selenium, copper, iodine, manganese, molybdenum, chromium, and fluoride.

A varied, well-balanced diet will provide your child with all the minerals he requires. Overdoses from mineral supplements can be very dangerous; always discuss supplements with your pediatrician before giving them to your youngster.

Calcium

The major component of bones and teeth, calcium is especially important during early childhood, when the skeleton and teeth are growing rapidly. Calcium is also important in maintaining a balance of body fluids, in the development of the nerves and muscle cells, and in blood clotting; in addition, it makes the absorption of vitamin B_{12} possible.

Daily Recommendations
Birth to 6 months: 360 milligrams
6 to 12 months: 540 milligrams
1 to 6 years: 800 milligrams
Sources
Dairy products, canned sardines and salmon with bones, nuts, legumes, dark green leafy vegetables.

Chloride

Like potassium and sodium (*opposite*), chloride regulates body fluids. It aids digestion by activating enzymes in saliva and in the stomach.

Daily Recommendations
Birth to 6 months: 275 to 700 milligrams
6 to 12 months: 400 to 1,200 milligrams
1 to 3 years: 500 to 1,500 milligrams
4 to 6 years: 700 to 2,100 milligrams
Sources
Table salt, meat, milk, eggs.

Chromium

A mineral about whose nutritive effects only a little is yet known, chromium apparently assists the body in the metabolism of sugars in foods.

Daily Recommendations
Birth to 6 months: .01 to .04 milligrams
6 to 12 months: .02 to .06 milligrams
1 to 3 years: .02 to .08 milligrams
4 to 6 years: .03 to .12 milligrams
Sources
Meats, cheeses, whole-grain breads and cereals, dried beans, peanuts, brewers' yeast.

Copper

Together with iron, copper helps form hemoglobin, the protein in the red blood cells that carries oxygen from the lungs to cells throughout the body. Full-term babies are usually born with adequate stores of the mineral; premature babies, however, frequently require supplements. Copper deficiencies are extremely rare but may result in anemia and a failure to thrive.

Daily Recommendations
Birth to 6 months: .5 to .7 milligrams
6 to 12 months: .7 to 1.0 milligrams
1 to 3 years: 1.0 to 1.5 milligrams
4 to 6 years: 1.5 to 2.0 milligrams
Sources

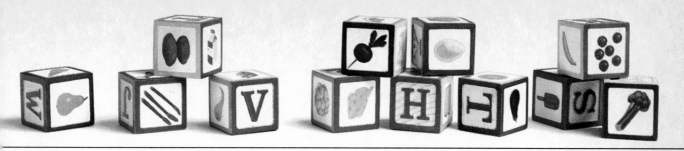

Organ meat, meat, poultry, nuts, whole grains, eggs, legumes.

Fluoride

As a builder of strong teeth, fluoride is often added to drinking water. A fluoride deficiency can cause tooth decay and, possibly, a weakening of bones in later years.

Daily Recommendations
Birth to 6 months: .1 to .5 milligrams
6 to 12 months: .2 to 1.0 milligrams
1 to 3 years: .5 to 1.5 milligrams
4 to 6 years: 1.0 to 2.5 milligrams

Sources
Seafood, foods grown with or cooked in fluoridated water, fluoridated water itself.

Iodine

Required by the body in minuscule amounts only, iodine is an essential component of thyroid hormones, which regulate metabolism.

Daily Recommendations
Birth to 6 months: 40 micrograms
6 to 12 months: 50 micrograms
1 to 3 years: 70 micrograms
4 to 6 years: 90 micrograms

Sources
Seafood, iodized table salt, sea salt.

Iron

This trace mineral helps form hemoglobin. Iron is also indispensable to the development of new muscle tissue and assists the body in resisting infection. Most infants are born with a three- to six-month reserve of iron. When nourished on breast milk or iron-fortified infant formulas, babies will get enough iron to prevent depletion of the reserve for up to six months; at the end of this period, the addition of solids to the diet ensures them new sources of the mineral.

Daily Recommendations
Birth to 6 months: 10 milligrams
6 months to 3 years: 15 milligrams
4 to 6 years: 10 milligrams

Sources
Liver, red meat, egg yolks, dried fruit, whole-grain or enriched breads and cereals, potatoes, legumes, leafy greens.

Magnesium

In addition to contributing to the bone-building process, magnesium transmits nerve impulses, regulates the body's temperature, and releases the energy contained in food into the system.

Daily Recommendations

Birth to 6 months: 50 milligrams
6 to 12 months: 70 milligrams
1 to 3 years: 150 milligrams
4 to 6 years: 200 milligrams

Sources
Meat, fish, and poultry, whole-grain breads and cereals, nuts and seeds, dark green leafy vegetables.

Manganese

Manganese is needed for good bone structure and a well-functioning nervous system.

Daily Recommendations
Birth to 6 months: .5 to .7 milligrams
6 to 12 months: .7 to 1.0 milligrams
1 to 3 years: 1.0 to 1.5 milligrams
4 to 6 years: 1.5 to 2.0 milligrams

Sources
Wheat germ, fruits, oatmeal, nuts, brown rice, legumes, whole-grain cereals, green leafy vegetables.

Molybdenum

Molybdenum is important in hemoglobin formation.

Daily Recommendations
Birth to 6 months: .03 to .06 milligrams
6 to 12 months: .04 to .08 milligrams
1 to 3 years: .05 to .10 milligrams
4 to 6 years: .06 to .15 milligrams

Sources
Whole grains, legumes, liver, kidney, dark green leafy vegetables.

Phosphorus

Necessary for good bone growth and other bodily functions, phosphorus is absorbed into the body with the aid of vitamin D. Because phosphorus occurs in so many foods, deficiencies of the mineral in children are unusual.

Daily Recommendations
Birth to 6 months: 240 milligrams
6 to 12 months: 360 milligrams
1 to 6 years: 800 milligrams

Sources
Meat, poultry, fish, dairy products, egg yolks, legumes, whole-grain cereals and breads, peanuts, tofu.

Potassium

In alliance with sodium, potassium helps regulate the amount and balance of body fluids. It also facilitates the contraction of muscles, the transmission of nerve impulses, and the release of energy within the body.

Daily Recommendations
Birth to 6 months: 350 to 925 milligrams

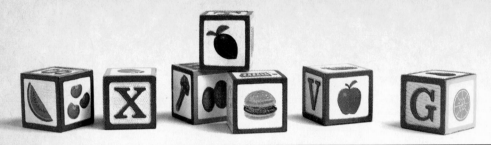

6 to 12 months: 425 to 1,275 milligrams
1 to 3 years: 550 to 1,650 milligrams
4 to 6 years: 775 to 2,325 milligrams
Sources
All fruits and vegetables.

Selenium

Like vitamin E, selenium prevents rapid oxidation or burning of
fat and vitamin A.
Daily Recommendations
Birth to 6 months: .01 to .04 milligrams
6 to 12 months: .02 to .06 milligrams
1 to 3 years: .02 to .08 milligrams
4 to 6 years: .03 to .12 milligrams
Sources
Seafood, liver, meat, poultry, egg yolks, whole-grain cereals and
breads, milk, garlic.

Sodium

Although sodium, found in salt and many foods, is needed for a
proper balance of fluids in the body and for various bodily
functions, most people, including children, consume far more of it
than necessary. Part of the problem is the excessive salt used in
many processed foods and the failure of most people to limit their
salt intake. Excess sodium can actually be harmful; it may cause
fluid retention in the body and contribute to high blood pressure.
Still, many parents, hoping to stimulate their child's appetite,
include salt unnecessarily in the dishes they prepare for him. Watch
your child's sodium intake; enough is present in milk, vegetables,
breads, and other foods to meet his daily needs.
Daily Recommendations
Birth to 6 months: 115 to 350 milligrams
6 to 12 months: 250 to 750 milligrams
1 to 3 years: 325 to 975 milligrams
4 to 6 years: 450 to 1,350 milligrams
Sources
Table salt, meat, poultry, fish, some vegetables such as celery and
Swiss chard, milk, eggs.

Zinc

Besides being a component of approximately a hundred enzymes
that facilitate chemical processes in the body, zinc is essential for
cell growth. Moreover, it helps store and transmit genetic
information within the cells.
Daily Recommendations
Birth to 6 months: 3 milligrams
6 to 12 months: 5 milligrams
1 to 6 years: 10 milligrams
Sources
Meat, liver, eggs, poultry, seafood, milk, whole grains, nuts, cheese.

When Good Nutrition Counts Most of All

A youngster's need for a nutritious diet begins in the womb, long before he is born. By eating properly, a mother-to-be lessens the risks of complications during pregnancy and delivery, and readies her body for the demands put upon it by nursing. And by making sure that she and her child get the steady supply of calories and nutrients they both must have in adequate supply, she lays the foundation for a well-nourished childhood and enhances his chances of growing up healthy and strong.

On the following pages are tips that will not only help you to select the foods that will be right for you and your baby during pregnancy and the breast-feeding period afterward, but also those that will be best for your little one as he grows from infant into active toddler and preschooler.

The pregnant mother's nutritional needs

During pregnancy, you eat for two, and your nutritional requirements naturally increase. The only way of ensuring that you get all the nourishment you must have is to eat a balanced diet (*page 46*). Because of protein's vital role in building tissue, you should consume at least seventy-five grams of pure protein daily, or a little over two-and-a-half ounces, which translates into about 300 grams of a protein food such as meat or eggs.

The building of a new human being demands that you have greater amounts of vitamins and minerals, also. To ensure that

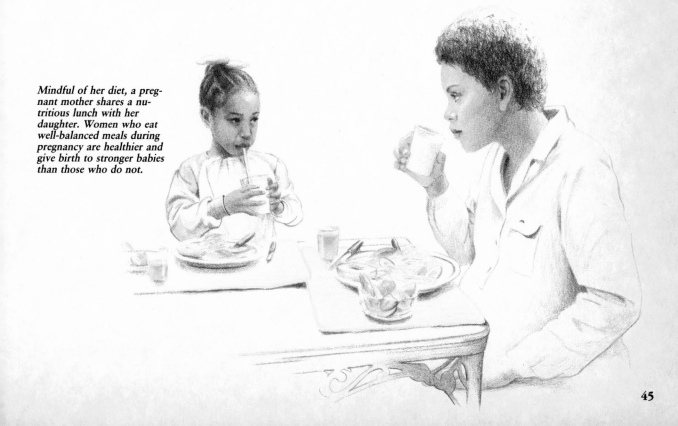

Mindful of her diet, a pregnant mother shares a nutritious lunch with her daughter. Women who eat well-balanced meals during pregnancy are healthier and give birth to stronger babies than those who do not.

Daily Foods for Pregnant and Nursing Women

Pregnant women and breast-feeding mothers have special nutritional needs. The chart below is designed to help you plan meals using recommended portions from the major food groups. In addition to foods such as these, you should consume six or more eight-ounce glasses of water or other caffeine-free drinks daily.

Food Group	Serving Size	Daily Servings	Key Nutrients Supplied
Meat and Meat Substitutes		Three (Four, if nursing)	Fat, iron, protein, phosphorus, vitamin B_1 (thiamin), vitamin B_3 (niacin)
Lean meat, fish, poultry	2–3 oz.		
Eggs	2 whole		
Nuts	1/2 cup		
Peanut butter	1/4 cup		
Legumes	1 cup		
Tofu	1 cup		
Milk and Milk Products		Four (Five, if nursing)	Calcium, carbohydrates, fat, phosphorus, vitamin A, vitamin B_2 (riboflavin), vitamin D, water
Milk (whole, low-fat, skim) or buttermilk	1 cup		
Cheese	1 1/2 oz.		
Yogurt	1 cup		
Cottage cheese	1 cup		
Fruits and Vegetables		Four	B vitamins, carbohydrates, folic acid, vitamin A, vitamin C, water
Vitamin C sources (citrus fruits and juices, berries, melons, mangoes, tomatoes, broccoli, cabbage)	1/2–1 cup	One or more	
Vitamin A sources (dark green and yellow fruits and vegetables, including peaches, carrots, spinach, squash, sweet potatoes, peas)	1/2–1 cup	One or more	
Other fruits and vegetables (including apples, bananas, potatoes)	1/2–1 cup	Two or more	
Breads and Cereals		Four	Carbohydrates, iron, protein, vitamin B_1 (thiamin), vitamin B_3 (niacin), zinc
Whole-grain or enriched breads	1 slice		
Ready-to-eat dry cereals	3/4 cup		
Cooked cereals	1/2 cup		
Rice, noodles, pasta	1/2 cup		
Whole-grain or enriched rolls or muffins	1 whole		
Crackers	4 whole		
Bagels	1/2		
Fats, Sugars, and Other Foods		No amount recommended	Carbohydrates, fats
Butter, margarine	1 tbsp.		
Mayonnaise	1 tbsp.		
Vegetable oil	1 tbsp.		
Salad dressing	1 tbsp.		
Sour cream	1 tbsp.		
Olives	5 small		
Pudding	1/2 cup		
Ice cream or ice milk	1 cup		
Cookies	2–3 medium size		
Cake	1 oz.		
Pie	1 1/2 oz.		
Sugar, honey, jam, jelly	2 tbsp.		

your baby develops strong bones, you should increase your calcium consumption by half and double your vitamin D intake. You can do so by drinking a quart of milk a day. Because your blood volume increases while you are carrying your child, you should increase the amount of iron in your diet as well, to about 60 milligrams daily. This can be accomplished by eating more red meat, liver, apricots, and dark green leafy vegetables. In addition, you need one-third more vitamin C, which you can get easily enough by drinking the equivalent of one cup of orange or grapefruit juice every day. You also need twice as much folic acid, a vitamin essential to the formation of DNA and RNA, the genetic code material present in every cell. It occurs in meats and such vegetables as spinach, peas, and broccoli.

Many pregnant women who make a point of eating wisely and well cut down on salt, fearing that sodium will cause water retention. Medical thinking on the issue has shifted, and salt-free or low-sodium diets are no longer recommended. This is because a woman's increased volume of blood during the nine months she carries a child actually amplifies her need for sodium.

Should you take supplements? Some doctors recommend vitamin and mineral supplements as insurance against nutrient deficiencies during pregnancy. Since it may not be possible to get iron and folic acid in sufficient quantities from your diet, these may be prescribed. Never take supplements of any kind without your doctor's approval; they can be toxic to your unborn baby. High dosages of vitamins A and D, for example, can produce birth defects.

A time for extra calories When pregnant, you should not just eat well but more. Ideally, you should gain two to four pounds during the first three months of your pregnancy and almost a pound per week thereafter — for a total gain of about twenty-five pounds. For most mothers-to-be, that means upping daily caloric intake by 300 calories, from a prepregnancy level of 1,600 to 2,400 calories to between 1,900 and 2,700. You can supply the extra calories easily enough by choosing calorie-rich items from the basic food groups.

Gaining fewer than twenty-five pounds may result in an underweight baby, who is more likely to experience medical problems early in life. But gaining over twenty-five pounds — even as much as forty-five pounds — should not be harmful to the child. However, any sudden gain should be reported to the doctor. A pregnant woman concerned about weight should never take off extra pounds unless advised to do so by her physician. She needs calories to ensure that her baby will be born healthy and strong.

Foods to avoid
A growing fetus is extremely vulnerable to hazardous substances that can be absorbed into the mother's body and passed to the baby. You should thus stay away from foods or drugs that contain potentially harmful contaminating chemicals. Make a point of reading food labels carefully (*page 63*) and of avoiding foods containing potentially carcinogenic colorings or artificial sweeteners. You will probably also want to abstain from alcohol and reduce caffeine intake during pregnancy. Large quantities of alcohol can restrict a baby's weight and cause developmental and learning disabilities. Caffeine, of course, lurks in many beverages besides coffee, including some soft drinks and cocoa, and you may decide to eliminate these, too.

A few words of warning
Throughout your pregnancy, eat safely as well as carefully. Stay away from raw or undercooked meats and raw seafood. Be extra cautious, too, about how you treat and store cooked or uncooked foods. Cover and refrigerate all leftovers. And be meticulously clean in preparing food, washing your hands before and after touching it, and making sure to scrub work surfaces.

Diet for nursing mothers
A nursing mother's diet influences not only the quality of her milk, but its quantity as well. Women who breast-feed should go on eating the same nutritious foods they ate during pregnancy (*page 46*), but in larger quantities, because their nutritional needs are now even greater. Naturally, since you are producing milk, you will need extra liquids. Consume two to three quarts of fluid a day, including at least one quart of milk. There is no evidence that moderate use of alcohol or caffeine is harmful during lactation, but it may be wise all the same to continue to limit consumption, as each can find its way into breast milk and thus into the baby. Caffeine may make an infant jittery, and alcohol will act as a sedative.

Most of the extra calories necessary for milk production come from your diet. Depending upon your baby's weight during her first three months of life, you may have to consume five hundred more calories a day than you did before you became pregnant. If your baby is older than three months and still nursing, you may have to up that amount to six hundred calories.

The newborn's diet
As a general rule during your baby's first year, you can expect her weight to triple and her length to increase by 50 percent.

As a result of this rapid growth, her nutrient and caloric needs will be greater per pound now than at any other time in her life. Breast milk is the ideal food for this period, containing all the water, protein, carbohydrates, fat, and basic vitamins and minerals (except vitamin D, iron, and fluoride) that your infant needs.

When is enough? A common worry among nursing mothers is that their babies are not getting sufficient nourishment. But most breast-fed infants easily receive the forty to sixty calories per pound of body weight that they must have each day. Be sure to nurse your baby whenever she seems hungry; your milk-production will regulate itself accordingly. As long as your baby is increasing in weight and generally seems content and happy, her breast-milk diet is probably supplying all the calories and nutrients she needs.

Formula feeding If you choose not to nurse your baby, commercial infant formulas will provide a completely nutritious diet during a baby's first six months. Most producers of formulas simulate breast milk by modifying cow's milk; the protein is lowered, vegetable fats and carbohydrates are added, and the entire mixture is fortified with vitamins and minerals. For those few babies who are allergic to cow's milk, nutritious formulas based on soy milk or cow's milk chemically predigested to rid it of allergens have been developed.

Formulas can be bought as liquids, or in concentrated or powdered forms to which water must be added. It is important to follow the directions carefully when storing and mixing a formula to guard against contamination.

The second six months By the age of six months, almost all babies have the neuromuscular control to swallow solid foods and drink from a cup. They can absorb proteins, fats, and carbohydrates better now, and their intestinal tracts have developed defense mechanisms against allergic reactions. By this age, too, most babies need the more concentrated form of calories and nutrients found in solid foods.

Weaning from breast and bottle Make the weaning process as gradual as possible; it will be less upsetting to your baby and, if you are breast-feeding, less uncomfortable for you. Because babies have an urge to suckle until they are at least one year old, most doctors recommend against weaning a baby completely until she has reached that age. If you stop breast-feeding before your child's first birthday, wean her to bottled formula before starting her on solids so

Keys to Healthful Eating

This chart specifies the daily number of servings from different food groups and the quantities in which items from each group should be served to provide children between the ages of one and six with the nutrients they need for proper growth. (*Box, page 105.*)

Food Group	Serving Size 1–3 years	4–6 years	Daily Servings	Key Nutrients Supplied
Meat and Meat Substitutes			Two or more	Fat, iron, phosphorus, protein, vitamin B$_1$ (thiamin), vitamin B$_2$ (riboflavin), vitamin B$_3$ (niacin), vitamin B$_{12}$ (cobalamin), zinc
Lean meat, fish, and poultry	2–3 tbsp.	2–3 oz.		
Eggs	1 whole	1 whole		
Peanut butter	1–2 tbsp.	2–3 tbsp.		
Legumes	1/4 cup	1/2–3/4 cup		
Milk and Milk Products			Four	Calcium, carbohydrates, fat, phosphorus, protein, vitamin A, vitamin B$_2$ (riboflavin), vitamin D, water
Milk (whole for children under two; whole, low-fat, or skim for children over two)	1/2–3/4 cup	3/4–1 cup		
Cheese	1 oz.	3/4–1 1/2 oz.		
Cottage cheese	1/2 cup	3/4–1 cup		
Yogurt	1/2 cup	3/4–1 cup		
Fruits and Vegetables			Four or more	B vitamins, carbohydrates, folic acid, iron, vitamin A, vitamin C, water
Vitamin C sources (citrus fruits and juices, melons, tomatoes, broccoli, cabbage)	1/2 cup	1/2–1 cup	One or more	
Vitamin A sources (dark green and yellow fruits and vegetables, including peaches, carrots, spinach, sweet potatoes, peas)	1/4 cup	1/4 cup	One or more	
Other fruits and vegetables (including apples, bananas, potatoes)	2–3 tbsp.	1/2 cup	Two or more	
Breads and Cereals			Four or more	Carbohydrates, iron, protein, vitamin B$_1$ (thiamin), vitamin B$_3$ (niacin), zinc
Whole-grain or enriched breads	1/2–1 slice	1–2 slices		
Ready-to-eat dry cereals	1/2–3/4 cup	1 cup		
Cooked cereals, rice, and pasta	2–4 tbsp.	1/2 cup		
Fats, Sugars, and Other Foods			No amount recommended (Use as needed for calories, but in moderation, with three servings maximum.)	Carbohydrates, fats
Butter, margarine	1 tbsp.	1–2 tbsp.		
Vegetable oil	1 tbsp.	1–2 tbsp.		
Mayonnaise	1 tbsp.	1–2 tbsp.		
Pudding	1/2 cup	1/2 cup		
Ice cream, ice milk	1 cup	1 cup		
Cookies	2–3 medium	2–3 medium		
Cake	1 oz.	1 oz.		
Pie	1 1/2 oz.	1 1/2oz.		
Sugar, honey, jam, jelly	2 tbsp.	2 tbsp.		

How big should a serving size be? Here, portions for a toddler and a preschooler come to roughly one-fourth and one-half of an adult portion. The extra half slice of bread for the preschooler ensures enough carbohydrates for her activity level and lets her use the protein in her diet for growth.

Preschooler portion

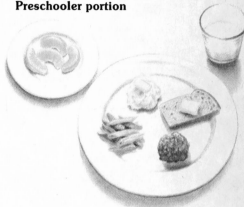

Toddler portion

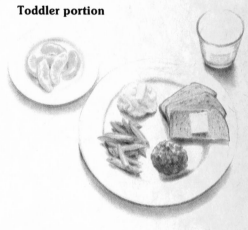

Adult portion

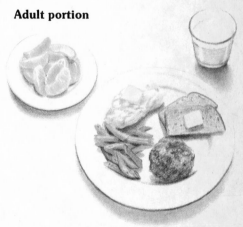

that she can continue to suckle. Do not give her unmodified cow's milk until she is getting at least two-thirds of her calories from solid foods. Drinking large amounts of cow's milk sometimes causes anemia when babies fill up on it and fail to eat other foods. Also, consuming more than one quart a day of cow's milk can lead to bleeding in the intestines, resulting in an iron loss. In fact, many doctors advise against introducing cow's milk until a baby is drinking regularly from a cup.

A nutritious first food

Fortified baby cereals, which are easy to digest and unlikely to cause allergies, make a good choice for a baby's first solid food. Many doctors urge that a baby be started on a bland rice cereal first because it is least likely to cause food-intolerance problems (*pages 66-75*). Mix the cereal with a little formula or breast milk, place a small amount on the tip of a spoon, slide it into your young one's mouth, and allow her to suck on it. After she has eaten about one or two tablespoons, let her finish her meal with bottle or breast. As the days pass, gradually increase the amount of cereal in her diet and cut down on mother's milk or formula.

When your baby is comfortably eating four to six tablespoons of rice cereal at each feeding, she is ready for another grain cereal, such as oats or barley, and eventually other solid foods, such as pureed fruits, vegetables, and meats. They should be introduced, however, one at a time. You can, of course, purchase these foods in jars at your local supermarket, or you can make them at home in a food mill, blender, or food processor (*page 104*).

Getting enough iron

By the time a baby is three to six months old, the stores of iron he was born with will have begun to diminish and his iron requirement will now have increased to about fifteen milligrams a day. Fortified baby cereals can supply the extra iron, and you should continue to give him these until he is two years of age. If you prefer to feed him nonfortified whole-grain cereals, such as rolled oats or brown rice, you may have to provide another source of iron, such as meat, liver, or apricots.

Caloric requirements of toddlers

Once your child has passed his first birthday, his growth will slow to about half the pace of his first year. As a result of this, his calorie demand will diminish somewhat, although he will continue to need regular supplies of nutrients. Most toddlers between the ages of one and three should consume about thirty-five to forty calories each day for every pound of their body weight. The calories should come from foods that are rich in vitamins and minerals, especially iron, calcium, zinc, and vitamins A, C, and B_6. Dairy products, meats, whole grains, and citrus fruits are the best sources of these.

The role of milk in a toddler's diet

Since homogenized cow's milk contains almost all the calcium, vitamin D, and B_2 (riboflavin) a growing child needs, it should be an important part of the toddler's diet. Give your youngster whole milk or properly diluted evaporated milk until the age of two; avoid skim or low-fat milks, which lack essential fatty acids and do not contain a sufficient number of calories. After he reaches two years, offer him whole, low-fat, or skim milk. A one- to three-year-old requires only about two or three cups a day, and if he eats other dairy products, such as yogurt or cheese, he will more than satisfy his need for the nutrients found in whole milk.

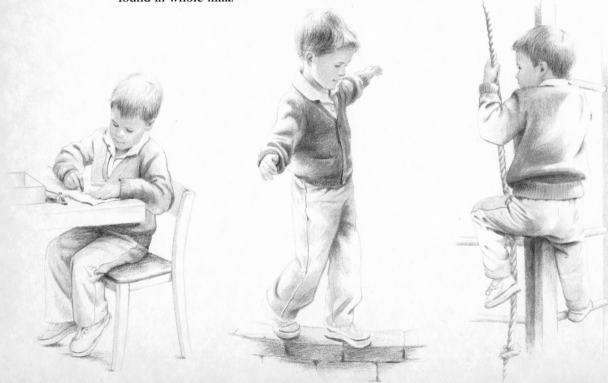

The child who dislikes milk   While some children drink too much milk, thus ruining their appetites for other foods, others refuse to drink it at all. If the child is not eating other calcium-rich foods, a calcium deficiency can result. Your reluctant milk-drinker should be encouraged to eat cheese and yogurt, or you can try sneaking liquid or powdered milk into the breads, puddings, pancakes, and hot cereals that he enjoys. Nuts, such legumes as peas and beans, and green leafy vegetables are also sources of calcium.

The preschool years   A preschooler's diet should be similar to that of her parents, providing they are eating a balanced diet, but with portions one-half to two-thirds as large (*page 51*). During the years three to six, your child's energy requirements per pound of body weight will decrease. But children in this age group still need plenty of nutrients and calories — about twenty to thirty-five calories per pound per day. The American Academy of Pediatrics recommends that children over the age of two — like adults — have a diet in which their fat intake is restricted to 30 to 35 percent of their total calories.

Be moderate in offering your child salty foods so as not to condition her to a high-salt diet. Watch your child's consumption of commercially prepared foods, most of which are high in sodium. As for sugar, enough of it exists naturally in foods, especially fruits, to meet all your child's needs. Although children have an innate preference for sweet foods, and yours is no exception, they should be taught the joys of eating nonsweet foods. ❖

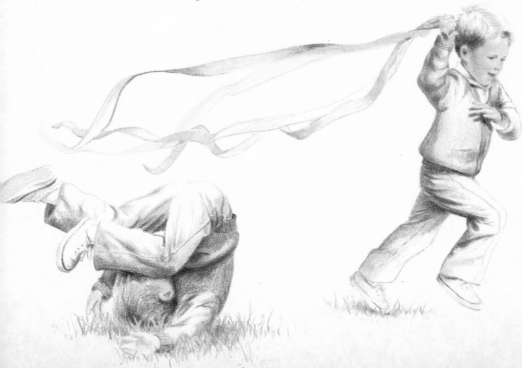

A whirlwind of motion, this energetic preschooler will burn up more calories each day than a less active youngster. Parents should encourage their children to get plenty of exercise and feed them a balanced diet to meet their energy needs.

Creating a Balanced Diet

Since eating habits are established early in life, it is important that you get your child enjoying healthful food from the start. Feeding him a nutritionally sound diet is not all that complicated, although it will require some planning.

Variety—the key
The best way to ensure that your youngster receives a well-balanced diet and gets all the nutrients and fiber he needs is to fix meals every day that contain foods from each of the four basic food groups: fruits and vegetables; milk and milk products; meat and meat substitutes; and breads and grain products (*page 50*). In building his diet from these four groups, strive to limit his intake of fat and of foods in which sugar is a major ingredient.

As background to your menu planning, keep in mind that there is no single food that your child must eat. If he hates peas, do not force him to eat them unless you want a struggle. Let him get the essential nutrients peas offer from other foods. If he loves peas, make sure he eats other vegetables, too. He should have not only a variety of foods, but a variety from each food group, especially fruits and vegetables, since these contain greatly differing amounts of individual nutrients.

A daily food plan
Nutritionists recommend that children between one and six years of age eat two or more servings of meat or meat substitutes every day, along with four servings of milk or other milk products, four or more servings of fruits and vegetables, and four or more servings of cereals and grains. To determine serving size, follow the rule of thumb that allows one measuring tablespoon of cooked food for each year of your child's life. This scheme, however, can only make an approximation of portion size since youngsters grow at different rates, and their appetites are constantly changing as their growth rate speeds up or slows down. Also, the more active a child is, the greater her need for calories will be.

Offering healthful snacks
There is nothing wrong with supplying nutritious foods at times other than breakfast, lunch, and dinner. In fact, the stomachs of youngsters are not big enough to hold food for several hours at a stretch, and they rarely can eat enough in three meals to satisfy their caloric and nutritional needs. So children must snack. As a concerned parent, you will want to make sure that the snacks you provide are packed with goodness, not merely sources of empty calories. And the best guarantee of healthful snacking is to keep only appropriate foods around the house (*pages 58–59*).

Vegetarian diets   A vegetarian diet can be as healthful for your child as one that includes meat if you are careful to include in each meal a meat substitute as a source of high-quality protein. Grains, legumes, seeds, nuts, and vegetables are all protein sources, but eaten alone they lack sufficient amounts of one or more of the essential amino acids required by a growing child. For a plant protein to be fully nutritious, it must be combined with another plant protein. Thus legumes, such as dried beans, soybeans, or peas, should be served with grains, such as wheat, rice, or corn. Still, to be safe, you would be wise to also include milk, cheese, and eggs in your child's diet since, like meat, they contain high-quality protein, as well as calcium and iron.

A strict vegetarian diet, excluding all animal protein, or one that fails to combine plant proteins properly can lead to serious physical and mental problems in small children, including anemia, growth failure, and irreversible brain damage.

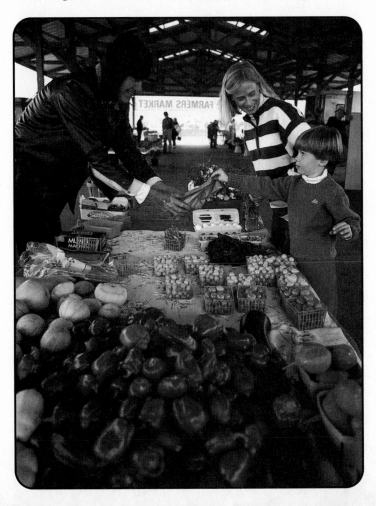

Curtailing sodium   Excessive salt in a daily diet over many years can produce high blood pressure in adults. One-third of all Americans suffer from the condition, which is the cause of many heart attacks and strokes. You can help your child avoid this health risk by getting her accustomed to low-salt foods while she is young. If you can prevent her from acquiring a taste for salt early in life, chances are she will not use it heavily as an adult. The best way to do so is never to add salt to your baby's pureed foods or cereals and to avoid serving your older child highly salted snacks. When buying processed foods, look for no-sodium or low-sodium brands. It is a fact that more than half of all the salt eaten by Americans comes hidden in processed foods.

Make a special effort to reduce the amount of salt you use in your cooking or, better yet, eliminate it altogether. Substitute lemon or lime juice, onion and garlic powders, and herbs and spices. And keep the salt shaker off the dinner table. Your child's sodium needs will easily be met by the sodium that occurs naturally in vegetables and dairy products.

Limiting saturated fat   Just as you may want to limit the salt in your child's diet, so you may also want to restrict the saturated fat. This is the villain in the buildup of cholesterol in arteries, which can lead to heart attacks. Remember, however, that a child should not be put on a relatively low-fat diet until his second birthday; during his first two years of life, he needs his food packed with calories to support his rapid growth.

When it is time, you can cut the fat in his diet by switching from whole milk to skim or low-fat milk. As for keeping fat consumption down further, serve him low-fat cottage cheese or cheese made with skim milk instead of hard or processed cheese. When buying meat, select lean cuts and trim off excess fat before cooking them. As an alternative to red meat, buy poultry or fish often. Be sure, however, to remove chicken and other poultry skin, since it contains high amounts of fat. Substitute chicken hot dogs and sandwich meats made from turkey for regular hot dogs and luncheon meats. Some brands of turkey bologna have one-third less fat than beef bologna, and some turkey salamis have one-fourth less fat than beef salami. When cooking, use a polyunsaturated vegetable oil, such as safflower or sunflower oil, in place of butter, lard, or solid vegetable shortenings. You can cook with margarine, but be sure the brand you use is high in polyunsaturated oil. Read the label; the first ingredient should be a liquid polyunsaturated vegetable oil rather than a "partially hydrogenated" or "hardened" oil. When cooking meat, choose broiling or baking when possible, since these let the fat drip off. Avoid frying.

Also, beware of fats hidden in processed foods. Read food labels carefully and steer clear of products that contain coconut oil, palm oil, or lard. Some manufacturers just list "vegetable oil" on their products without saying which one; stay away from such items, for the oil may be highly saturated.

Cutting down on sugar

Sugar is an empty calorie food. Although it contains only sixteen calories a teaspoon, it has nothing else to offer. For this reason, and the fact that sugar is a cause of tooth decay, you should restrict the amount your child eats. Do not stock your kitchen with cookies and sugar-coated cereals. Instead, serve fresh fruits for dessert and unsugared whole-grain cereals sprinkled with fresh or dried fruit for breakfast. Offer your child sweets as an occasional treat — a cake on his birthday or homemade caramel apples at Halloween — but do not make them a part of his daily diet. Never reward him with cookies, candies, or desserts, and encourage your friends and relatives to refrain from giving him these.

Sugar is present in many foods. A tablespoon of catsup may hide up to a teaspoon of sugar. Two tablespoons of peanut butter can include one to two teaspoons, and a cup of fruit-flavored low-fat yogurt can contain more than four teaspoons. Figuring out the amount present in a product is not always easy. Although ingredients must be listed in order of predominance on the label, food manufacturers can confuse shoppers by listing different kinds of sugar. Be alert for the following on labels: corn syrup, corn sweetener, honey, sorghum, dextrin, and words ending in *ose* — sucrose, lactose, maltose, dextrose, and fructose. All are types of sugar.

Fast foods

Most youngsters love eating at fast-food restaurants, and in today's busy world, parents often find it convenient — despite the nutritional drawbacks. The problem with these foods is not what they lack, but what they contain — too much sodium and too many calories supplied by fat. But if most of your child's meals are well-balanced, you have no need to feel quilty over an occasional visit. A typical fast-food meal of fried chicken with a roll or of a hamburger, french fries, and a shake does include three of the four major food groups, and if you add lettuce and tomato or a salad, the fourth group, fruits and vegetables, is also represented.

Because the chicken and fish are deep fried, there is little to

Targeting Your Child's Foods

One way to ensure a wholesome diet for your child is to think of your daily food choices as targets on a dart board. As in a game of darts, your aim should be directed at the bull's-eye (*opposite*), where a sampling of foods high in nutrients are found. But you can also score nutritional points, albeit in lesser amounts, by hitting areas farther from the center. Remember, there is no single food that a child must eat to be healthy. Your goal simply is to make sure that your youngster eats a varied, balanced diet. (Items that are inappropriate for a child younger than two are discussed on page 105.)

Ideally, the foods listed in the bull's-eye should make up the backbone of that diet. They include whole-grain breads and cereals, fresh vegetables and fruits, poultry, lean meats,

fish, milk, and low-fat milk products. They can be eaten anytime, including snacktime (*below*). They have been targeted because they are rich sources of protein, carbohydrates, dietary fiber, polyunsaturated fat, vitamins A, B_2 (riboflavin), and B_3 (niacin), iron, and calcium.

The ring immediately around the bull's-eye includes a sampling of foods that are more heavily processed or higher in saturated fat than the target foods. Finally, the outer circle includes highly processed convenience foods and sweets. These generally contain fewer nutrients than those items lying closer to the bull's-eye or are high in fat, added sugar, or salt. No parent should aim to make them a part of her child's daily diet, but no harm will come if your youngster eats them in small portions every now and then.

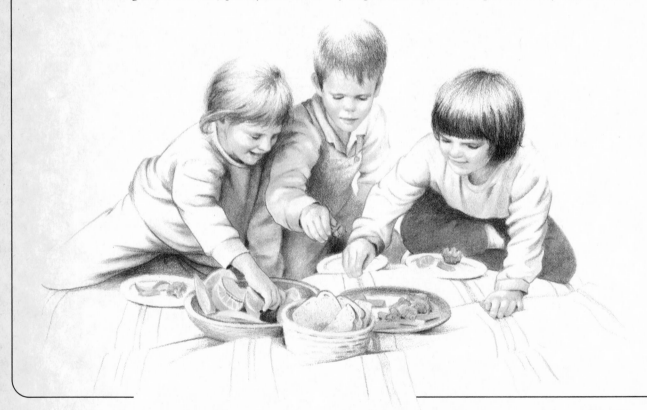

At a pretend picnic, these preschoolers dive into a snack of un-buttered whole-wheat bread, bananas, apples, oranges, and raw carrots and broccoli — healthful foods from the center of the target at right.

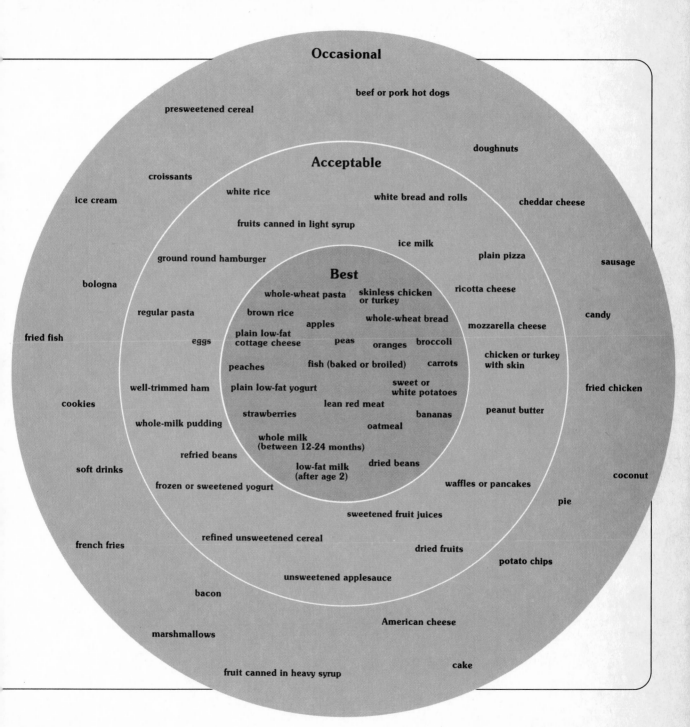

Occasional

beef or pork hot dogs

presweetened cereal

doughnuts

Acceptable

croissants

white rice

white bread and rolls

cheddar cheese

ice cream

fruits canned in light syrup

ice milk

plain pizza

sausage

ground round hamburger

Best

bologna

whole-wheat pasta

skinless chicken or turkey

ricotta cheese

candy

regular pasta

brown rice

whole-wheat bread

mozzarella cheese

apples

fried fish

eggs

plain low-fat cottage cheese

peas

oranges

broccoli

chicken or turkey with skin

fish (baked or broiled)

peaches

carrots

fried chicken

well-trimmed ham

plain low-fat yogurt

sweet or white potatoes

cookies

lean red meat

bananas

peanut butter

strawberries

whole-milk pudding

oatmeal

whole milk (between 12-24 months)

refried beans

dried beans

soft drinks

low-fat milk (after age 2)

coconut

frozen or sweetened yogurt

waffles or pancakes

pie

sweetened fruit juices

french fries

refined unsweetened cereal

dried fruits

potato chips

unsweetened applesauce

bacon

American cheese

marshmallows

cake

fruit canned in heavy syrup

59

choose between them and a hamburger in terms of fat content. But whichever one your child orders, do not allow her to pour on the accompanying sauces; these add empty calories and unwanted sodium. If she orders fried chicken, before she takes her first bite, remove as much of the skin as you can to lower the fat content. Your best bet is pizza, provided you stay clear of the traditional meat toppings, which can be fatty and salty. Plain cheese pizza or pizza with a vegetable topping has only about 25 percent of its calories in fat. Also, the tomato sauce provides vitamins A and C, the cheese protein and calcium, and the crust various B vitamins.

As a beverage, a milk shake is a better choice than a soda. Although loaded with sugar, fast-food shakes do have nutritional value; some are fortified with iron, and most contain significant amounts of protein, calcium, vitamin B_2 (riboflavin), and niacin. Of course, plain milk or water is better still.

Whole foods vs processed foods

Fresh and minimally processed foods are generally more nutritious than foods that have been highly processed. Fresh fruits and vegetables, for example, have slightly more vitamins and minerals than their canned counterparts. Frozen produce, on the other hand, keeps more of its nutrients intact. Indeed, if the freezing is done immediately after picking, frozen fruits and vegetables can often be better for you than fresh produce that has been sitting on a supermarket shelf for a few days.

Whole-wheat or rye breads, graham crackers, and brown rice are more nutritious than white breads made with refined flour and are an important source of fiber. Whole-wheat flour contains five times more niacin and three times more iron than white flour. This is because it is ground from the whole-wheat berry, including the berry's nutrient-rich outer layer, or bran, and the tiny part of its inner kernel, called the germ. In milling white flour, these parts are eliminated — together with up to 80 percent of the berry's noncaloric nutrients and much of its fiber. To make up the loss, white breads are enriched, a process that returns some nutrients, but not the fiber.

Thus, it is wise to accustom your child to the taste of bread, pasta, rice dishes, and other foods made from whole grain. When purchasing bread, look for the listing of "100 percent whole wheat" or another whole grain as the first ingredient. Do not be fooled by the color; many manufacturers call their products wheat bread when in fact they have merely added caramel coloring or molasses to make them look more beneficial than they really are.

Whole grains

You can add interest to your child's diet by varying the types of grains you serve her. Besides whole wheat, let her sample such tasty grains as buckwheat and oatmeal or a grain preparation such as bulgur, which is cracked wheat.

Natural and organic foods

Be wary of the claim that a food is "natural." Often the designation is there simply because the food manufacturer has found it helps to sell the product. In fact, being natural is not necessarily synonymous with being healthful. Natural foods are usually defined as foods that have no artificial ingredients. But manufacturers often put the label on products that contain preservatives, emulsifiers, and high levels of salt, fat, and sugar. Remember, too, that the designation does not necessarily mean that the foods are harmless. Coconut, a common ingredient in granola cereals, for example, is high in saturated fat; and the honey found in "natural" soft drinks still leads to tooth decay.

The term *organic* tends to be misused less often, but you should still be wary of any label carrying it. Organic fruits, vegetables, and grains are grown in soil enriched with animal manures, humus, compost, or residues or extracts from other organically grown foods, rather than with commercial fertilizers. No pesticides, herbicides, or fungicides are used. Organic meat and dairy products come only from animals that have been raised on natural feeds and that have not been treated with antibiotics or hormones.

Because organic foods are supposedly free of potentially dangerous man-made chemicals, some food experts recommend that consumers buy them whenever possible. Unfortunately, they often cost two or three times more, and you cannot always be sure that what you are purchasing is truly chemical-

With his dad's guidance, a five-year-old helps himself to the salad bar at a fast-food restaurant. Wise food choices — here, hamburger, bun, low-fat milk, lettuce, and tomato — can nutritionally enhance a fast-food meal.

free. There are no guarantees that potentially harmful pesticide residues may not have run off from other areas and found their way into the grower's land. Some plants contain naturally occurring toxins, and some may be contaminated by natural fertilizers. If you do want to feed your child organic produce, your best bet is to grow your own or purchase it directly from a reputable grower at your local farmers' market. Food cooperatives, which usually buy organic food through growers' associations and sell in cost-saving bulk quantities, are another good source for you to consider.

Food additives

Additives are substances food manufacturers put into their products to enhance their appearance, texture, or flavor, or to keep them fresh until they reach your table. In some food products, additives replace vitamins and minerals that have been lost during processing, or they provide nutrients that were not there originally. The addition of iron to baby formula and to bread, for example, has made everyone healthier.

Some additives are natural products derived from plants. Lecithin, a fatty substance found in soybeans and used as an emulsifier in processed foods, is one. Other additives are manufactured. Among these are ascorbic acid, which is synthetic vitamin C, and beta carotene, the orange color found in carrots, which the body can convert into vitamin A. Still others, such as saccharin and butylated hydroxyanisole, or BHA, a preservative that prevents fats from becoming rancid, are synthetics in their own right.

Additives to avoid

Although most food additives are perfectly safe, some scientists have expressed concern about a few of the synthetic ones — most notably, artificial colorings; brominated vegetable oil (BVO), an emulsifier and clouding element in some citrus-flavored soft drinks; monosodium glutamate (MSG), a flavor enhancer commonly used in soups, seafood, and poultry; saccharin, a noncaloric sweetener; and sodium nitrates and nitrites, the preservative and coloring agents found in smoked fish, bacon, ham, and luncheon meats. Studies have linked these chemicals to cancer and other health problems in animals. Until the final word is in, be wary of foods that contain them.

The best way to cut down on the amount of additives in your child's diet is to avoid heavily processed food and to keep soft drinks, which are loaded with additives, out of the house. Search for brands made without additives or prepare more of these foods from scratch at home (*pages 98-137*). ❖

How to Read a Nutrition Label

The U.S. Food and Drug Administration requires manufacturers to place nutrition labels on certain products, including foods for special dietary use, foods to which nutrients have been added, and foods advertised with specific nutrient claims. The labels appear in the standard format shown below. Key nutrients are always listed in the same order and in metric measures. The symbol *g* stands for gram (28 grams equal 1 ounce), *mg* for milligram (1,000 milligrams equal 1 gram), and *mcg* for microgram (1,000 micrograms equal 1 milligram). Individual servings, which the labels also provide, are often recorded in ounces or cup measures.

When comparing brands for nutritional value, check the serving sizes given on the labels. A brand that appears to offer more of a particular nutrient, such as protein, may in fact have only a larger serving size.

By law, nutrition labels must state not only the size of an individual serving, but also the number of servings per container, the number of calories, and the number of grams of protein, carbohydrate, fat, and sodium contained in a serving. In addition, the labels may provide optional information about the percentages of saturated and polyunsaturated fat in the product, the different kinds of carbohydrates present, as well as the amount of cholesterol contained. Label amounts are based on averages; the actual amounts may vary by as much as 20 percent. If a food is ordinarily eaten with another food, such as dry cereal with milk, the nutritional information for the combination of these foods is often given.

```
NUTRITION INFORMATION
       (per serving)

     serving size = x oz.

  servings per container = x


calories . . . . . . . . . . . . xxx

protein . . . . . . . . . . . . . x g

carbohydrate . . . . . . . . x g

fat . . . . . . . . . . . . . . . . . x g

sodium . . . . . . . . . . . . . x mg


     PERCENTAGE OF U.S.

        RECOMMENDED

     DAILY ALLOWANCES

          (U.S. RDAs)


protein . . . . . . . . . . . . . . x %

vitamin A . . . . . . . . . . . . x %

vitamin C . . . . . . . . . . . . x %

vitamin B₁ (thiamin) . . x %

vitamin B₂ (riboflavin) . x %

vitamin B₃ (niacin) . . . x %

calcium . . . . . . . . . . . . . x %

iron . . . . . . . . . . . . . . . . x %


  INGREDIENTS: additives,

artificial color, artificial flavor, or

      optional ingredients,

  preservatives and their purpose.
```

The U.S. Recommended Daily Allowances are the amounts of protein, vitamins, and minerals that the average individual requires to remain healthy. Nutrition labels list the U.S. RDAs by percentage. In a healthful diet, the intake from all sources of each nutrient should reach about 100 percent daily. The nutrients listed here must appear on labels; other nutrients may be included at the manufacturer's option.

Ingredients are listed by weight. Specific quantities are not required and variations of the same ingredient may be included. Sugar sources, for example, may be listed several times under other names, such as dextrose or lactose. All additives, including artificial flavors and preservatives, must be identified. Since many common foods, such as jellies, pasta, and tomato products, conform to standard recipes agreed to by both the FDA and the manufacturer, the ingredients need not be listed on the label. But if the manufacturer changes the recipe, the ingredients must be listed. Many manufacturers, on a voluntary basis, regularly include them.

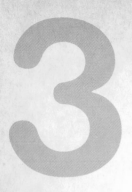

When Food Is Cause for Concern

There are times in almost any youngster's life when her eating habits will change or must be altered. A child who has a cold or fever, for example, will probably not feel up to regular meals and will want to be coddled with a soothing diet until her health returns. Fortunately, such an interruption in a child's normal eating habits rarely demands more than a week's repertoire of special foods.

Other conditions, however, such as food allergies and intolerances, can entail long-term changes in the child's daily fare. And a number of chronic ailments are dramatically affected by what a child eats. In these instances, it is usually necessary to exclude some foods from a youngster's diet and to find nourishing substitutes. When a child's problem is overweight, on the other hand, you may not need to eliminate any one item but simply to balance carefully all the foods you prepare and monitor serving portions.

Modifying a child's diet in any of these ways invariably takes some extra thought and effort. You may, for example, find it necessary to screen packaged or processed foods for hidden allergens or irritants, as the mother and daughter on the opposite page are doing. Nevertheless, dietary restrictions need not cause family tension or make a child unhappy. Although she may not like missing out on foods others can have, you can give her loving support and include her in the process of planning and watching her diet. When you use this approach, she will very likely develop a sense of pride in taking good care of herself.

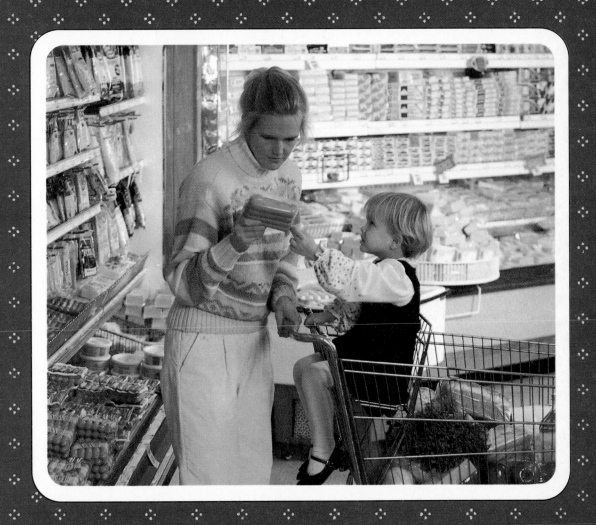

Those Mysterious Food Sensitivities

Physical reactions to food often present themselves in a confusing fashion. Symptoms may not be limited to the digestive system; indeed, they may occur anywhere in the body apparently without relationship to the diet. As a consequence, by the time a youngster is eating a number of different foods, it can take some real detective work first to identify the problem as a dietary one and then to discover which food item is causing the irritation.

It is, however, well worth the effort needed to track down a suspected food sensitivity, as anyone can tell you whose child has had the benefit of a proper diagnosis. If the symptoms turn out to be nonfood related, you will then be in a position to look for other causes. But if they are food linked, you will have the satisfaction of seeing your little one's good health and spirits restored as soon as you modify her diet.

Kinds of food sensitivities Although food sensitivities are of many types, most of them fall into two broad categories. Those that involve the immune system are true allergies. Those that do not — and this includes many different kinds of reactions to food — are generally known as intolerances.

The mechanism of a food allergy is fairly well understood. Substances in a food — allergens — pass from the child's digestive tract into his bloodstream. There, they trigger the production of antibodies, which on subsequent exposure to the food cause varying kinds of physical distress, a true allergic reaction. But why some children have such reactions to foods that do not affect other youngsters is unclear. Among several possible causes under investigation are an imbalance in the immune system and a problem with the digestive tract itself, which permits substances that should be contained in the intestines to pass into the bloodstream.

Since a baby's digestive tract needs time to mature, you should be particularly cautious about introducing your infant to foods that are likely to cause allergies, such as eggs, wheat, and peanut butter. Scientists believe that a tendency to manifest allergic reactions is probably inherited. The infant or child may or may not inherit the same allergy as the parent, but simply the allergic predisposition. On a somewhat brighter note, most scientists also agree that true food allergies are uncommon in adults as well as children.

Intolerances — or nonallergic reactions — are more common, but they still are probably not as widespread as some people think. Like allergies, they seem to be tied to the genetic

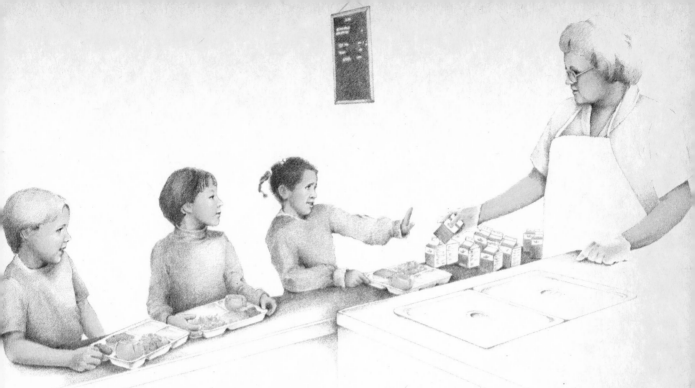

code in one way or another. Some of the best understood of these conditions are triggered by a deficiency of enzymes in the body. The lactose-intolerant child, for example, may have an insufficient supply of the enzyme that is needed for the proper digestion of lactose, the sugar in milk. Or the youngster may lack the enzyme entirely.

Other food sensitivities may manifest themselves in quirky reactions to substances that do not adversely affect most youngsters — food additives, for example, or naturally occurring chemicals, such as caffeine in iced tea. It is more than likely that such reactions have a biochemical basis also, but one that has yet to be identified.

Food intolerances can be psychological as well as physical. For instance, if a child becomes ill after eating a particular food, her association of that item with the way she felt at the time may lead her to feel nauseated the next time she eats it, despite the fact that her original illness was caused not by the food, but by a virus or even by stress. Although her response to the item is a product of her mind only, it nevertheless continues to be very real to her. If your child reacts this way to a certain food, do not force her to eat it.

Common symptoms

The symptoms of food sensitivities are as diverse as their causes. Most frequently, the affected child will suffer some kind of digestive upset — a stomachache, abdominal bloating, diarrhea, vomiting. But both allergies and intolerances can produce symptoms in other parts of the body as well. The skin may be affected, flushing or breaking out in hives; the lips, eyes, and throat may swell; or the child may have respiratory distress

Signaling no, a kindergartner declines the milk offered in her school's cafeteria. A digestive intolerance to milk has helped teach her to take responsibility for her own diet.

67

— a runny nose, a cough, a wheeze — usually accompanied by digestive or skin reactions.

In addition, symptoms may range in severity, from a mild syndrome to an acute response in which the youngster has difficulty breathing and may even lapse into unconsciousness. Any extreme reaction requires emergency medical treatment — usually a shot of Adrenaline®. Parents of children who have had a life-threatening reaction to food should — under their doctor's direction — keep a medical kit on hand containing an Adrenaline®-loaded syringe that can be purchased in a drug-store and used at a moment's notice. Severe reactions like this — which, fortunately, are rare — tend to be allergic and almost always occur within minutes of the time an allergen has been ingested. Less acute reactions may manifest themselves some hours later. This lag in time can make it difficult for parents to ascertain whether the symptoms that appear are the result of their youngster's having eaten a particular food or whether they have another origin.

Problem foods

All the same, there are a number of foods to which small children can have genuine adverse reactions of the allergic type. Among the most common culprits are cow's milk, eggs, corn, wheat, peanut butter, and soy, which crop up unexpect-edly in many foods (*box, opposite*). Fish, shellfish, and nuts can also trigger reactions, often quite severe in nature. Berries give rise to troublesome symptoms in some small children; it is wise therefore to wait until a youngster is a year old before introducing these foods.

Diagnosing food sensitivities

If your child displays any of the symptoms that are described here, you should consult your pediatrician, who will assess the child's health and outline procedures for you to follow. You will need to identify the offending food, a process of careful observation and trial-and-error experimentation. Many parents keep a food diary, cataloging everything their youngster eats. You may want to do the same, as well as keep track of any symptoms your little one develops, maintaining a record of their onset and severity.

You will be told to eliminate a suspect food from your child's diet for a few weeks. Most children will not be harmed by following a restricted diet for a short time, and if a particular item proves to be indeed at fault, your youngster's symptoms should begin to disappear fairly rapidly after the food has been eliminated from his diet. Once they do, if you have cut out

Hidden Allergens

Wheat, eggs, milk, soy, and corn are the most common triggering agents of food allergies in children younger than three. They crop up in products under varying names. Anyone who has a child who is allergic to these foods should check the labels on all commercially prepared and packaged foods to determine whether they contain any of the possible allergens. Some products in which they may occur are listed below.

WHEAT
• Commercial baby foods; processed cheese; luncheon meats; hot dogs; canned meat products; hamburger extenders; frozen meat and fish products; bottled salad dressings; bottled or powdered sauces and gravies; canned or powdered soups. In checking labels, avoid products containing wheat gluten, gluten flour, hydrolyzed vegetable proteins, durum wheat flour, bran, farina, graham flour, malt, and monosodium glutamate (MSG), which is sometimes made from wheat.

EGGS
• Bottled salad dressings and garnishes; baked goods and pastries; powdered cake and dessert mixes; and canned or powdered soups and sauces. Egg white may be listed on labels as albumin or ovalbumin. It is frequently used as a glaze on baked goods and candies. Eggs may also be used to produce lecithin, an emulsifying agent found in a wide variety of foods.

MILK
• Many baked goods, breads and pastries; creamed canned and powdered soups; bottled or powdered sauces; milk chocolate; mashed potato mixes; and bottled salad dressings. Milk may be found on ingredient labels listed as casein, lactalbumin, globulin, lactoglobulin, powdered milk solids, and sodium caseinate.

SOY
• Tamari sauce; miso; tofu and tofu-based products; commercial baby foods; cereals; baked goods and pastries; powdered cake and dessert mixes; some cheeses; commercially prepared and powdered dip mixes; nondairy milk substitutes; drink mixes; ice cream and ice cream cones; puddings; candy; frozen meat and fish products; hamburger extenders; luncheon meats; some pastas; corn chips and potato chips; bottled salad dressings; mayonnaise; shortening, oil, and margarine; and canned and frozen vegetables. Soy is commonly used in the production of the emulsifying agent lecithin.

CORN
• Hominy grits; maize; some vegetable starches and vegetable broths; canned baby foods; frozen desserts; powdered cake and dessert mixes; baking powder; carbonated drinks; malted drinks; bleached wheat flour; chewing gum; cereals; canned and frozen soups, fruits and vegetables; syrups; jams and jellies; margarine; luncheon meats; rice mixes; bottled salad dressings; monosodium glutamate (MSG); seasoned salt; Tabasco® sauce; some vinegars; Worcestershire sauce; tortillas; and peanut butter and nuts roasted in vegetable oil. Corn oil may be included in vegetable oils and shortenings without being identified on the label. Corn syrup may turn up as an ingredient in candies and baked goods as a sweetener.

---

several foods, you will need to test further in order to see which one produces the reaction.

Finding the cause In order to determine which food is the culprit, reintroduce one by one the items that you cut out of your child's diet. Doctors refer to this as the food challenge. Keep the portions small at first; then gradually increase them, either until the symptoms reappear or until the child is eating her usual amount without any reactions. If, for example, orange juice is one of the foods that has been excluded from your youngster's diet, you might give her a couple of sips the first day of the experiment, an ounce or two the second, and half a glass the third. Wait five days before trying the next food to be sure no symptoms appear in the meantime. Anytime her symptoms recur, of course, you will want to stop serving her the irritating item. If the symptoms disappear after you do so, you have probably identified at least one of the sources of your little one's difficulties.

Further tests Your child's physician may want to confirm any positive responses, since previous bad experiences with a food can affect the youngster's reaction to it and even the way a parent interprets his response. In the doctor's office or a clinic, the child will be given a small amount of the suspect food in disguised form — mixed into applesauce, for example. If he reacts after the suspect food has been given to him without his knowledge, the diagnosis is almost certain.

When the sensitivity seems to be allergic in nature, the doctor may also want to perform a skin test in order to confirm the diagnosis and to recommend treatment. As with skin tests for other allergies, the youngster's forearm or back is pricked or punctured with a needle using an extract of the food allergen being tested. If the extract causes a welt of a certain size to form, the youngster is more than likely allergic to that food. However, it is often necessary to confirm the positive skin test by another carefully done food challenge. Here the proof of the pudding is literally in the eating.

Coping with food sensitivities

Often, prescribing the cure for a food sensitivity is easier than implementing it. For one thing, you need to eliminate the offending foods from your little one's diet, and this is often hard to do. It requires reading food labels carefully to be certain that a processed product does not contain the very item you are seeking to avoid.

When a staple, such as milk or wheat, is implicated, you will have to modify not only what you offer your child to drink or eat, but also some of your recipes. Fortunately, there are a number of cookbooks on the market containing recipes designed for people with various allergies and intolerances. And health-food stores are usually well stocked with goods for the food-sensitive youngster.

As long as your child is still a small baby, you should have little trouble making sure the foods she eats are safe for her, since you are almost always the one to make up her menu. And anytime she is cared for by a relative or baby-sitter, you will be able to leave clear instructions about what she may and may not be given to eat.

Eventually, however, your little one's horizons will broaden, and you will have to take a few more precautions to keep her diet free of harmful foods. You will want to alert adults at her nursery school or day-care center, as well as the parents of any children with whom she plays. There is no need to make a fuss over the issue; if you address it in a matter-of-fact way, so will everyone else.

For special occasions, such as a friend's birthday party, you may wish to pack a special treat for your youngster to bring along with her, just in case something is served that she should not have; or you can deliver it in advance so that the host mother is able to present it with a minimum of fuss. And when you eat out at a restaurant with your child, make sure you know what is in each dish—if necessary, bring along food you know is safe for her to eat.

Most important, you will want to help your child to assume some of the responsibility for managing her own diet. Explain the condition to her as soon as you think she can understand and tell her that there are other children who must avoid certain foods as well. Be matter of fact. Do not complain about the extra work it is causing you. At the same time, do not offer her pity. Simply tell her, "This food makes you sick, so you should be careful never to eat it. That's too bad, but there are many other delicious things you can eat." And name some of them. Take her shopping with you for the foods she enjoys and have her help prepare some of her special dishes at home. If you accept the problem and help your little one to handle it, she will not feel that she has been singled out to face an unfair hardship. It can be useful, too, to have the whole family share the child's diet in the beginning, until she adjusts to her restrictions.

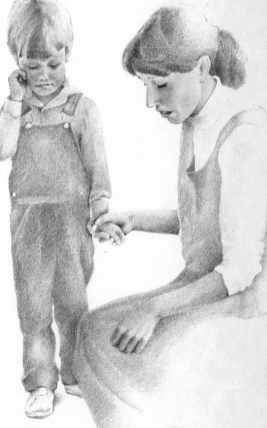

Scratching the itchy rash that has broken out on his face, a boy gazes at its cause as his mother explains again that he is allergic to chocolate and must not eat it.

Preventing allergies   Experts recommend several ways to minimize a youngster's chances of developing a food allergy or intolerance. For newborns, some studies indicate that breast-feeding is preferable to bottle-feeding, since breast milk introduces fewer foreign proteins into the infant's delicate digestive system. However, it is well to recognize that the minute amounts of proteins obtained from the mother's diet and present in her milk may be sufficient to stimulate a food allergy in the infant. Hence, the breast-feeding mother should avoid ingesting foods of high allergic potential.

Whether the baby is breast- or bottle-fed, she should not be given any solid food until she is at least four months old. Even then, it should be introduced slowly, one item at a time, with a three-day wait between each new food to see how the baby reacts to each.

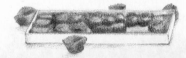

Once the child is eating a number of different foods, she should be given a varied diet. Too much of any one food at a time, or the same item on the menu for several days in a row, just might trigger a food sensitivity in a small child. Serving different foods from day to day — within reason, of course — is considered the best way to determine which foods she will or will not tolerate.

Outgrowing food sensitivities Since children often outgrow food sensitivities, you can check later to see whether your child still reacts to the item that earlier gave her a problem. Unless she has had a severe reaction to a food, or your physician has advised you otherwise, give her the item about six months after you first removed it from her diet. Start with a small serving — perhaps just half a teaspoonful. Assuming she has no adverse reaction this time, increase the amount progressively over the next few days. If she begins to manifest her old symptoms, eliminate the food, but try it six months later. If she has no adverse reaction, she has probably outgrown the problem. Happily, most food sensitivities disappear before the child enters first grade; probably due in part to the maturation of the immune system. ❖

An Expert's View

Can Diet Cause Hyperactivity?

Hyperactivity, properly called attention deficit hyperactivity disorder, ADHD, is a diagnostic label applied to about 5 percent of American school children who are unusually active, restless, or aggressive, with poor impulse control, a short attention span, and a decreased tolerance for frustration.

Because of the subtle distinction between hyperactivity and a young child's normal energy, hyperactivity may be very much in the eye of the beholder. Studies have shown that the label is used more often by older teachers, presumably because they have a lower tolerance for disruptive behavior. And the term is applied most often in wintertime, when children are cooped up indoors. Interestingly, the condition is five to ten times more common among boys than girls.

Of the many theories advanced to explain hyperactivity, one in particular has produced controversy. In 1973, Dr. Benjamin Feingold, a California pediatric allergist, proposed that hyperactivity is brought about by certain food ingredients — particularly naturally occurring salicylates (chemicals related to aspirin) and artificial colors and flavors. To treat hyperactivity, Dr. Feingold advocated a rigorous elimination diet that excluded most fruits, many vegetables, all commercially produced baked foods, luncheon meat, ice cream, powdered pudding, candy, soft drinks, tea, coffee, margarine, colored butter, condiments, and many medicines.

Critics found Dr. Feingold's distinction between artificial and natural food ingredients quite arbitrary. Many laboratory-synthesized flavors are chemically identical to naturally occurring flavors, so there is no reason for a child to respond differently to the artificial flavor.

The Feingold diet has since been evaluated in several well-designed studies by pediatricians and behavioral scientists, who have not been able to substantiate the theory. When hyperactive children who previously had seemed to respond to the diet were unknowingly given an additive-containing diet in a double-blinded experiment, neither parents nor teachers could distinguish between the children's behavior on the two diets.

Most authorities today believe that the best treatment for truly hyperactive children involves behavior modification therapy and often medication.

When families ask me about the Feingold diet, I make my reservations clear, then let them try it if they wish. The Feingold theory has great appeal because it offers a simple solution to a complex problem. Some parents find it easier to blame the foods their child is eating than to consider other possibilities — that he may be behaviorally disturbed, perhaps, or that other problems cause his disruptive actions.

Do elimination diets harm the ADHD child? Perhaps. Restrictive diets increase the risk of poor nutrition, and they may give rise to neurotic attitudes toward food that will persist into a child's adult years. Thus, I would discourage exclusion diets of any kind.

—Elliot F. Ellis, M.D.
Chief, Allergy and Clinical Immunology
Nemours Children's Clinic, Jacksonville, Fla.

Special Medical Conditions Affected by Diet

Children sometimes have disorders that can be partially controlled through the foods they are served. These conditions range from the more common lactose intolerance to the rare celiac disease, whose victims are unable to digest gluten. Untreated, such disorders can cause serious side effects and in some cases even death. Fortunately, several of them that had grave consequences just a few decades ago are far better understood today. Modern testing techniques allow accurate diagnosis and careful monitoring, and special diets, often prescribed in conjunction with medicine, can help keep the disorders in check.

Lactose intolerance
In some children the inability to tolerate milk may be due to low levels of the enzyme lactase, which breaks down milk sugar, or lactose, so that it can be absorbed by the body. Most often lactase deficiency develops after a bout with an intestinal infection, in which case the problem may disappear after the child's intestine has fully healed.

Lactose intolerance, which occurs with some frequency among Asians, blacks, and peoples of Mediterranean origin, usually develops well after the baby's first year, most often around puberty, and gets worse with age. The symptoms are bloating, gas, cramps, and diarrhea. Since several tests exist for diagnosing the condition, you should consult your pediatrician if you think your little one suffers from lactose intolerance. Treatment varies with the severity of the disorder. A youngster who has some lactase may well be able to handle small amounts of milk at a time and perhaps some cultured milk products as well, such as yogurt. Most lactose-intolerant children can drink normal quantities of milk if the milk is mixed first with a widely available nonprescription lactase enzyme that breaks down lactose and makes it digestible. For severely intolerant children, there are low-lactose dairy products on the market; soy milk is an option.

Galactosemia
Another, far rarer, disorder that is associated with milk is known as galactosemia. In this inherited condition, galactose — a component of lactose — builds up in the body of the child. The disease, which has several forms, becomes evident within the first days or weeks when the baby drinks milk, whether it be his own mother's or the cow's milk that is used in a commercial baby formula. Symptoms of this disorder are vomiting, diarrhea, and weight loss. Many hospitals routinely test newborns for the ailment, since, left untreated, it can result in serious

liver damage, cataracts, mental retardation, and even death.

A child with galactosemia should be seen regularly by a physician and should avoid milk and milk products and medication with lactose fillers. Infants must be given a special formula that includes sufficient nutrients; toddlers and small children may need vitamin supplements also. In some cases, dietary restrictions can be relaxed slightly when the child is older, but the condition never goes away.

Phenylketonuria

All states require screening of newborns for phenylketonuria— or PKU—a potentially devastating disease transmitted by a recessive gene. Only about one newborn in 14,000 is affected, but untreated, the ailment leads to severe mental retardation. PKU babies lack the enzyme needed to metabolize phenylalanine, an essential amino acid in all proteins. Human and cow's milk contain phenylalanine.

If a blood test at birth reveals the disorder, the infant will be fed a special formula to limit her intake of the amino acid to just the amount necessary for normal growth and development. As she matures, she will be put on a low-protein diet rich in fruits, vegetables, and grains. She will require regular monitoring to keep her phenylalanine level in balance, and her diet will have to be adjusted to suit the changing needs of her growing body. Some experts believe the diet can be liberalized once the child's nervous system is fully formed. Still, any youngster with PKU will be obliged to adhere to a careful regimen for life.

Celiac disease

A small percentage of children are unable to digest gluten, a protein found in many grains, including wheat. Called celiac disease, this condition is probably partly genetic, although experts are not clear yet as to how it is inherited or exactly what process in the body triggers it. In those affected by the disease, gluten damages the intestines, inhibiting the absorption of fats and other nutrients. One symptom of the condition are loose, bulky, foul-smelling stools. Curiously, a child born with celiac disease develops tiny buttocks. He may also be slight for his age and suffer from muscle weakness.

The condition is serious, and you should consult a doctor if you suspect that your youngster has celiac disease. The remedy involves eliminating the gluten-containing grains — wheat, rye, barley, and oats — and substituting rice, corn, soy flour, and potato starch. After being put on the diet, children with the condition return to good health rapidly, providing they are not exposed to hidden sources of gluten in processed foods. (The ever-popular hot dog, for example, may conceal fillers that contain gluten.)

Cystic fibrosis Cystic fibrosis is a troubling, often fatal disease in which some gastrointestinal symptoms can be partially controlled through diet. Transmitted by a gene, it is the most common inherited recessive disorder among Caucasians in the United States — about one child in 2,000 is affected. The chief cause lies in the secretions of the digestive and respiratory tracts. Instead of producing a clear, thin liquid, the cells manufacture a thick mucus that eventually clogs ducts in the lungs, pancreas, and intestines. Symptoms, which usually appear during infancy, are weight loss despite a good appetite; a chronic cough as the child tries to expel the mucus, excessively salty sweat; and often, as in celiac disease, loose, bulky, foul-smelling stools, since fat is poorly digested.

For better nutrient absorption, the child should eat a diet relatively low in fats and relatively high in protein and carbohydrates. Vitamin and iron supplements and pancreatic digestive enzymes are usually prescribed as well. Together with other forms of treatment, this diet can ease the discomfort of cystic fibrosis and prolong the child's life.

Diabetes mellitus Diabetes mellitus — or insulin-dependent diabetes — is relatively rare in infants and toddlers; its onset usually takes place between the ages of five and seven or at puberty. It occurs because the pancreas, a gland located behind the stomach, stops producing insulin, a hormone that enables the body to utilize the energy-containing glucose manufactured from other carbohydrates. Without insulin to regulate it, glucose builds up in the youngster's bloodstream and her body begins to ransack its own muscles and fat for energy supplies. Symptoms are excessive hunger, thirst, and high urine production as well as weight loss and fatigue.

Frequently, the disease can be well controlled with a careful balance of daily insulin injections and diet. Most experts these days do not insist on particular foods, just a diet that is wholesome and nutritious. Meals and snacks should be served at regular times, and portions should remain consistent from one day to the next. In this way, the amount of glucose the body produces stays in balance with the daily insulin injection. This keeps the youngster in good health and minimizes damage to the arterial blood-vessel system, which is a potential complication of the disease.

Diets for Childhood Ailments

When your child is ill, he will need a suitable diet. Here are recommendations for a variety of conditions.

Colds and Coughs: A child with a respiratory infection can eat whatever he wants, although his low level of activity may subdue his appetite. Light, soothing foods, such as soups, puddings, and ice cream, are usually appealing to a child with a cold or sore throat. Encourage him to drink liquids of all sorts but be sure not to force them on him; he will consume as much as he needs.

Fever: A fever will cause your child to burn up more calories than she does when she is well. Still, do not fret if she refuses most food for the first day or two of her illness. She will probably be thirsty, however, so offer her something to drink every half hour of the waking day—fruit juice, nondiet soda, weak tea with sugar, water. As the youngster starts to feel better, her interest in food will pick up a bit, but she will probably prefer bland foods.

Vomiting: It is not uncommon for a child to vomit when ill, especially if she has a fever. After she has thrown up, avoid giving her anything to eat or drink for an hour or two to allow her stomach to recover. Then try a few sips of water or flat soda. If she can keep them down, wait fifteen or twenty minutes and offer her a bit more. Gradually increase the amount given at one time to about four ounces. Once a few hours have passed with no further vomiting, you can offer her bland foods. Should she vomit again, stop all foods and fluids; resume liquids after another resting period. If your child is not yet two, has kept nothing down for four hours, and is still vomiting, call your physician; such a young one can become dehydrated in just a few hours.

Diarrhea: Dehydration is also a major concern when a youngster has diarrhea. If the child is vomiting as well, the danger increases, and you should call the doctor at once. A physician should also be consulted if the child is under one year of age and appears to be losing weight. In general, though, if your youngster has diarrhea, give her plenty of fluids to replace what she loses each time she has a bowel movement. Infants should have about two ounces every four hours; preschoolers about half a cup. If the diarrhea is occurring only once every four to six hours, you can offer bland foods as well — rice cereal, dry toast, perhaps a mashed banana. Avoid giving other fruits or fruit juices until the child's stools are normal.

Hypoglycemia

Hypoglycemia stems from any one of nearly a dozen conditions that lower the level of glucose in the blood and are the cause of periodic attacks. Symptoms include pallor, sweating, irritability, listlessness, lack of coordination, and, in the worst instances, even convulsions and coma. If you suspect that your youngster may have hypoglycemia, you will need to take him to the doctor as soon as possible for diagnosis; if left untreated, the disorder can damage the developing central nervous system. Although it is rare during childhood, the condition is more common in newborns, especially those who are premature or have low birth weight. When it occurs during the early years, hypoglycemia is often caused by a liver-enzyme deficiency. A high-carbohydrate snack, given when early symptoms appear, is usually enough to ward off a full-scale attack. More frequent meals, containing adequate amounts of carbohydrates, are another effective preventive measure. And by the time the child is eight or nine years old, the condition will in all probability disappear entirely. ∴

Concerns about Weight—
How Realistic Are They?

Although it is natural to be concerned if your child seems unusually chubby or skinny, you should know that there is actually a broad range of acceptable weights for young children. Most thin youngsters, even those who seem to their parents to be all bones, are quite healthy. And usually, a fat baby will not grow up to be overly stout.

When obesity extends into the preschool years, however, it can become a problem. Studies show that about 25 percent of seriously overweight preschoolers will be fat later in life. And along with the burden of their pounds, obese adults tend to carry the weight of additional stress and health problems. Fortunately, in many cases, a youngster who begins life chubby will slim down naturally. Because childhood is a time of rapid growth, overweight boys and girls often do not need to lose pounds; all they have to do, in fact, is maintain a constant weight as increased height cancels excess pounds. And in the process the healthful eating habits they pick up from their parents will help them control their weight into adulthood.

In trying to decide whether your child has a weight problem, you should be aware first of what constitutes a normal growth pattern. Over the initial twelve months of her life, your youngster will gain pounds rapidly; indeed, she will roughly triple her birth weight. After this, she will gain more slowly — approximately five pounds a year until puberty, when the rate will again accelerate. Even so, a big increase in weight during her second year need not be viewed necessarily as abnormal. She is, for one thing, growing taller.

Once she passes her second birthday, however, your youngster's weight gains should be roughly similar to those of her peers. And in terms of the weight- to-height ratio (*charts, pages 78–79*), you should expect her to stay in approximately the same percentile from year to year.

Weighing a child — as this nurse is doing at an annual checkup — can reveal the effect of a balanced diet: a normal weight gain.

Causes of obesity   The basic physiological cause of obesity is no mystery: More energy, in the form of calories in food, is taken into the body than is burned up through activity, growth, and tissue repair. As a result, the body stores the unused energy in the form of fat.

No one truly understands, however, what causes some children to become fat while others, who may eat the same amount of food — or even more — do not. Genetic makeup seems to be one key factor; body build, for instance, which affects weight to a great extent, is largely inherited. And even the total number of fat cells a person develops is thought to be passed down in the genetic code. Study after study has shown that a child whose biological parents are obese is far more likely to be overweight than one with slim parents.

This does not mean, however, that a youngster with a genetic tendency for putting on weight must automatically become fat. Eating styles and habits are determinants, too, as is the child's activity level. Similarly, stress and unhappiness can affect a child's appetite, the anxious child turning to or away from food as the case may be.

Healthful eating habits   Healthful eating habits grow out of infant feeding practices and

A Weight-Height Chart: Where Does Your Child Fall?

Charting a child's weight and height together (a weight-to-height ratio) can help tell whether he has a weight problem. Use these graphs, adapted from National Center for Health Statistics growth charts, which show normal weight ranges for different heights.

First, you will need to measure and weigh your child. For a youngster under two, who cannot stand straight enough to be measured accurately, the measurement should be taken with the child lying down on his back. To obtain the weight, use an accurate spring scale. To use the graphs, measure your child and choose the graph appropriate to his sex and age. Find his height along the bottom of the graph and draw a verticle line from this point straight into the graph, through the colored curves. Next, find his weight along the left side of the graph and draw a horizontal line from there, extending it until it intersects with the vertical line. If the lines intersect within the colored curve, the child's weight-height ratio is in the normal range.

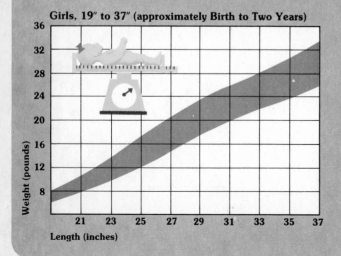

Girls, 19″ to 37″ (approximately Birth to Two Years)

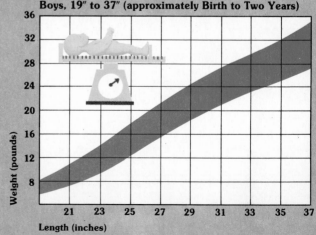

Boys, 19″ to 37″ (approximately Birth to Two Years)

are refined as the child begins to eat solid foods and joins the family for meals. From the beginning, you should yield to your youngster's indications that she has had enough to eat or drink. Never urge an infant to keep feeding, for example, if she has turned away from breast or bottle. Experts believe that even tiny babies have a precise instinct for their own nutritional needs. This instinct — or satiety signal — seems to be a complicated feedback mechanism in the brain. As long as you do not teach your child to override this signal, it should help her to regulate her eating habits throughout her life. Thus there is no need to pressure your youngster into finishing everything on her plate, especially if she says she is full.

Your role is to provide a balanced diet and to create an atmosphere that encourages judicious eating habits. Not only will you want to plan healthful meals and snacks, but to pay attention to portion size as well (*page 51*).

The overweight child If you have an offspring who puts on weight readily, include plenty of foods that he enjoys but give none of them in excess. Ask him about his preferences, and unless he names only potato chips and hot dogs, follow his suggestions as often as you can.

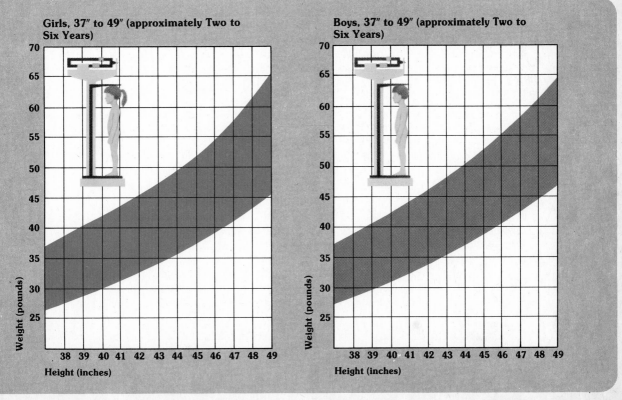

Girls, 37″ to 49″ (approximately Two to Six Years)

Boys, 37″ to 49″ (approximately Two to Six Years)

Seek to satisfy his appetite and cravings without indulging him. Try serving foods with a variety of textures—smooth and crunchy, soft and crisp. Chewy foods — meats, nuts, crusty breads — allay hunger especially well. You will want, of course, to estimate the fat content of the meats and nuts you give your child to make sure that he obtains no more than 35 percent of his calories for the day from fat. Include foods, too, that are high in bulk and low in calories, such as fruits and salads. If he begins meals with these items, the edge will be off his appetite when he gets to the higher-calorie courses. By the time the occasional dessert arrives, a small portion should do.

It is also helpful to serve meals and snacks at regular times. This not only encourages good eating habits; it also seems to moderate weight gain. Therefore, do not allow your child to nibble at odd hours or to go without a meal, only to make up for his hunger by giving him extralarge helpings at the next. Cutting calories drastically for any length of time is not wise, either: It slows the metabolism and makes shedding fat more difficult. And it can damage a growing body, too. Controlling portion size is a far better solution.

There are other ways you can help a youngster who is struggling with a weight problem. If you decide not to serve him dessert, for instance, be considerate and forgo serving one to the others at the table; studies show that it is easier for a child to thin down if the whole family shares his diet for a time. And do not leave tantalizing foods in accessible cupboards—or worse, out on counters. Finally, consider the beverages the youngster consumes. Low-fat milk, water, and small amounts of fruit juice are best for a child who is inclined to be plump.

Exercise is important

An increase in exercise can boost a child's metabolism as much as 30 percent, burning off unneeded calories. When coupled with sensible eating habits, regular exercise will help a child to keep his weight in check.

There are a number of ways to encourage a child to be active. To begin, be sure to give a baby plenty of space to wiggle and crawl about freely. And provide toys that elicit movement—balls, push-pull toys, wheeled vehicles. You can increase your little one's activity level by taking him on frequent walks, playing catch, or romping with him on the living-room floor.

Keeping food in perspective

A child who is fed wholesome foods when hungry, played with when in need of attention, and encouraged to be active when restless will more than likely develop a healthy attitude toward food. You need to observe your child carefully so you can distinguish genuine hunger from other needs. As much as you possibly can, avoid using food as a pacifier or bribe (*pages 25–27*).

If your little one is already too preoccupied with food and eats to meet other cravings, take a psychological approach and begin diverting his attention to new activities and outlets. Try to be sensitive to his moods — offer him hugs when he seems lonely, for example, and help him find a game to entertain him when he is at loose ends. By doing so, you will be showing him that he can be fulfilled without resorting to the comfort of food.

The underweight youngster

At the opposite extreme from the child who develops a double chin just looking at a brownie is the youngster who appears to be too thin. While this can be worrisome, most skinny children are actually quite robust. Nevertheless, if you are concerned about your child's thinness — or have noticed signs of another problem that may be keeping him from gaining weight — you should consult a doctor. At the very least, you will receive some professional reassurance. You can stimulate your youngster's appetite by supplying a wide variety of tempting foods. Serve him whole milk often, and whenever possible, use it in cooking. Remember also to make several healthful snacks available to him throughout the day.

Two youngsters walk home from the supermarket with their mother, instead of riding in the family car. Boosting a child's activity level burns off extra calories and helps prevent the buildup of fat.

Developing a positive attitude

Perhaps the most important thing to keep in mind is to accept your child as he is, however much or little he may weigh. Some children are just naturally skinny, others will always be overweight, no matter how much is done to adjust their food intake. In the long run, the child must learn to live with and like himself. He can do this only if you show him how. If he is fat, help him dress in a way that does not accentuate his condition; compliment him on his appearance. Offer positive reinforcement when he sticks to an eating plan but do not criticize him when he strays. Be generous with hugs and kisses and tell him that he is special to you just the way he is. ❖

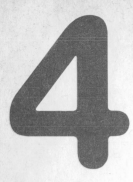

Good Times with Food

Cooking from time to time with your youngster can be one of the special pleasures of parenting. As you allow him to help, the bond between you and your little one can only expand and strengthen.

Yet there are many other reasons to involve your child in culinary activities. On the most basic level, cooking with your preschooler is an excellent way to teach him about good nutrition and about the origins of the foods he eats, something not readily apparent from the meat and poultry case or the vegetable bin at the supermarket. As the photograph opposite charmingly suggests, a child will also delight in trips to the country, where he can see things actually growing. He may even be able to enjoy the fun and satisfaction of harvesting food and then tasting it, learning about freshness in the process.

All his emerging skills — mental as well as physical — will be brought into play as he participates with you in preparing a meal or treat for the family. On the following pages, you will find a variety of suggestions for special trips and projects that will enhance your youngster's experience with and appreciation of food. You can start when he is quite young, a toddler, really, and though he may not quite rival a world-class chef by the time he is six, he will feel himself an increasingly competent little person with a fund of knowledge about food and its properties.

Imagine the boost to his sense of accomplishment and confidence when you serve a dish he has had a hand in cooking, and you give him a smile and a compliment. What is more, there is an important fringe benefit to it all: By learning about food and its preparation, he is bound to be more willing to sample and accept dishes that are new to him, and likely to enjoy his food more.

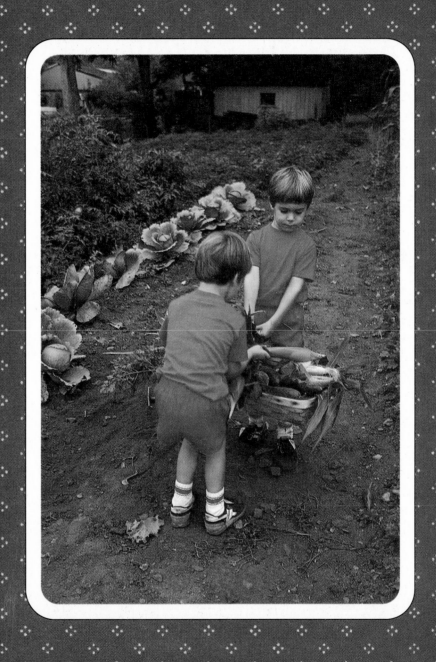

Learning through Cooking

Whether your child is peeling carrots or mashing potatoes, he is sure to be learning something interesting and useful by lending you a hand with your mealtime tasks. And he will find it all great fun. Every youngster loves to imitate adults, and your small helper will enjoy himself immensely as he practices adult skills. While he is at it, he will be learning about the special properties of the ingredients he is working with — the carrots' brilliant color and firm texture, and the way potatoes soften and become deliciously smooth when beaten with butter and milk. Indeed, there will be an education in practically everything you do together in the kitchen.

The language of cooking

Like most such endeavors, cooking has its own vocabulary. Inviting your youngster to help in the kitchen will introduce her to the fascinating language of foods and their flavors, of cooking utensils and techniques. And because your child is naturally building associations as she acquires new vocabulary, she is likely to remember the words and will know how to use them when she is outside the kitchen. When your young assistant licks her fingers after squeezing a lemon, she will truly understand the meaning of the word *sour*. And when she stirs gelatin into a bowl of water, she will be able to see precisely what the word *dissolve* means.

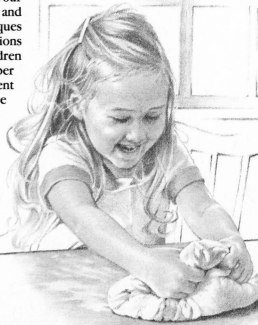

Kneading bread dough, a girl gets exercise while she has fun. Once the bread has risen, she can help put it in the oven and then join her mother in waiting for the first warm, crusty slice.

Yet building a vocabulary is only part of the experience. Preparing food together opens up many avenues for conversation between you and your child — discussions about what to make and who will do which tasks, followed by critiques of the finished products. These conversations may even range far from the kitchen; children are naturally curious, and your young helper most likely will want to know where different foods come from as well as how they are transported from one place to another.

And there is more. Preparing food can provide your preschooler with a splendid opportunity to practice prereading skills. Many dishes require recipes, and by kindergarten, your young cook will have the ability to work following a simple set of instructions — especially if you are willing to translate them into illustrations or diagrams. As a matter of fact, there are many well-illustrated books on the

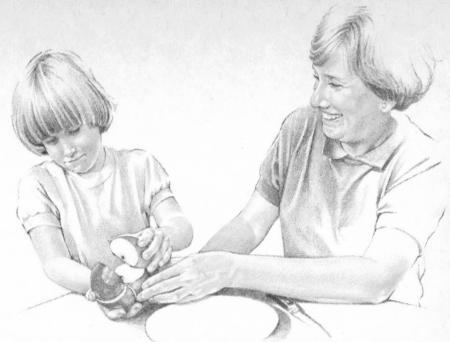

An explanation of fractions might be beyond this little girl, but not when her mother demonstrates the concept of quarters and halves by cutting up an apple into four equal parts.

market that are specifically designed to teach preschoolers as much as possible about foods, cooking, and the origins of various kitchen staples (*box, page 87*). When you read them aloud to her, such books are sure to reinforce the vocabulary your youngster has just learned at your side.

Sensory awareness and motor control

All children delight in exploring with their senses, and cooking is nothing if not a sensory experience. With only a little encouragement from you, your youngster will soon be fully engaged in an exciting examination of how food looks and tastes and smells. There are textures to explore, too — soft cookie dough and its transformation into the crisp cookies themselves — and even sounds to enjoy, such as popcorn popping and bacon sizzling.

Preparing food also helps develop your little one's motor skills. Rolling out a piecrust and kneading bread require the use of large muscles in the back and arms. Stirring and beating exercise the hand muscles, while cracking an egg provides your youngster with a chance to apply his fine-motor control. And nearly every kitchen task from pouring milk to buttering bread requires eye-hand coordination — which improves rapidly with practice.

Picking up math skills

Helping you in the kitchen provides your preschooler with another important benefit — training in a number of basic math skills. She practices counting and discovers fractions while measuring out ingredients, explores the concept of time while waiting for a cake to bake or bread dough to rise, and learns to make one-to-one correspondences by serving food — three dishes of pudding, for example, for three people. Her culinary efforts and her new experiences with kitchen equipment may bring her in touch with geometry, too, since she will be working with food and equipment of various sizes and shapes: Pans can be round or square; a peppercorn is tiny compared with a pineapple; a Christmas tree cookie cutter consists of triangles one on top of the other.

The science of cuisine

As every good cook knows, there is a considerable science to the preparation of food. Ingredients react in specific ways when they are combined, beaten, heated, or chilled. A small child may find much of it to be magical — a soufflé puffing up in the oven, cream turning to butter after it has been shaken long enough, or the transparent egg white becoming opaque when it is heated in the pan.

You can help your little one to understand that such changes are science, not alchemy, by providing simple explanations and showing him that foods react in predictable ways. This will demonstrate to him the overall principle of cause and effect, and he will learn an important life lesson — that each of his actions has a particular, often foreseeable result. In turn, this will help him acknowledge the world as a reasonably orderly place over which, however small he may be, he is able to have some control.

Food can broaden cultural horizons, as this boy is discovering by assembling a treat new to him — a Mexican taco.

There is yet another sense in which cooking will educate your youngster in the sciences. Since he will be working according to a recipe at least some of the time, he will be learning the virtue of following directions carefully, a skill that is necessary in successfully carrying out all manner of tasks in later life.

Creativity and imagination

Although it is important for your child to learn how to follow directions, it is also wise to let her experiment every once in a while, taking her cues from her own impulses. Art is as important as science to the culinary world, and out of mistakes have come some great discoveries. Moreover, as your youngster experiments, she learns that there is often more than one way to prepare a dish — and that can lead to another important lesson in life. Allowing your child to use her imagination when she cooks will encourage her to ap-

Books about Food to Share with Children

Story and Science Books:

The Apple and Other Fruits by Millicent Selsam.
Autumn Harvest by Alvin Tresselt.
Blueberries for Sal by Robert McCloskey.
The Boy, The Baker, The Miller and More adapted by Harold Bersen.
The Carrot Seed by Ruth Krauss.
Creative Food Experiences for Children by Mary Goodwin and Gerry Pollen.
Farm Morning by David McPhail.
From Seed to Pear by Ali Mitgutsch.
From Milk to Ice Cream by Ali Mitgutsch.
The Ginger Bread Boy by Paul Galdone.
The Great Big Enormous Turnip by Aleksei Tolstoi.
How Tevye Became a Milkman by Gabriel Lisowski.
I Like Fruit by Ethel Goldman.
Let's Grow a Garden by Gyo Fujikawa.

Let's Look Up Foods from Many Lands by Beverley Birch.
Mr. Rabbit and the Lovely Present by Charlotte Zolotow.
The Magic Porridge Pot by Paul Galdone.
More Potatoes! by Millicent Selsam.
Peanut by Millicent Selsam.
The Popcorn Book by Tomie DePaola.
Stone Soup (old Russian folk tale).
The Story of Johnny Appleseed by Aliki.
The Tale of Peter Rabbit by Beatrix Potter.

Cook Books:

Cook and Learn by Beverly Veitch and Thelma Harms.
Cooking with Kids by Caroline Ackerman.
Cup Cooking by Barbara Johnson and Betty Plemons.
Let's Bake Bread by Hannah Lyons-Johnson.
Love at First Bite by Jane Cooper.
More Than Graham Crackers by Nancy Wanamaker, Kristin Hearn, and Sherrill Richarz.

proach other situations creatively, looking at tasks and problems from several different angles before deciding on any one particular approach.

Your youngster's experiences with food are bound to enrich her other creative endeavors. It may add to her fantasy play; as she becomes familiar with what goes on in the kitchen, she will be able to fill in numerous details when she pretends to be a parent or a cook. And as she busies herself with cuisine, she is continually gaining fresh inspiration for her art projects. The colors of fruits and vegetables may inspire a still-life painting in dazzling hues or a collage based on pictures of food that she has cut from magazines.

Social and cultural values

Finally, your youngster stands to gain a number of positive social habits and attitudes from his adventures in the kitchen. Food has deep cultural significance, and by preparing a variety of foods, a youngster can explore his own heritage as well as that of others. For one thing, he can learn respect for people of different cultural backgrounds. Learning about diverse cuisines teaches him about the world beyond his immediate neighborhood. It also helps build his respect for differences among people. And if he is involved in preparing foods as ethnically diverse as burritos, blintzes, and crepes, he will see in them similarities as well as differences.

At the very least, as he cooks with you and others, he will be practicing such basic social skills as cooperation and taking turns. Along the way, he is likely to learn the value of patience, since foods that are cooked too briefly or mixed too rapidly rarely taste quite right. And he will almost certainly develop a healthy respect for the amount of work that goes into the preparation of a meal — which might just encourage him to use good table manners and to try dishes or foods that are new to him. Moreover, he will come to understand that cooking for another person can be one of the most satisfying ways of showing love and care. ∴

Where Foods Come From

When you look at the supermarket through your youngster's eyes, you will see that it can be a very misleading place. There, gathered in one huge room, is almost all the food the family eats. Everything is clean and orderly; most items are neatly packaged. There is not the least suggestion of the fields and orchards where produce grows, the open spaces where cattle roam, the hard work that goes into raising and processing foods. A child may reasonably conclude that the supermarket is where food "grows," just as he may imagine that there are little people inside a television set.

Helping your child learn about the origins of food is a natural complement to his adventures in the kitchen. You may live too far away from an orange grove to show him where his morning juice comes from — although you might make a point of visiting one while you are on vacation. But there are sure to be plenty of places at home where you can track supermarket items to their origin — be it the sea, the land, or a factory where foodstuffs are processed. The following section offers suggestions for a few such outings;

you will undoubtedly think of more as you and your youngster work together in the kitchen.

Going on Field Trips

The first thing your youngster will observe on your field trips is that all food comes from either the plant or the animal world. And she will go on to acquire a wealth of knowledge as she sees the many ways that foods are raised, harvested, and processed. You will want to arrange your trips in advance, making sure that small visitors are welcome, and that the place is not only appropriate but also safe, with enough supervision to keep youngsters from wandering into potentially dangerous areas. Spend some time talking with your youngster about the upcoming expedition. Reading her a book that relates to the trip will stimulate her curiosity and imagination. Once you are at your destination, help her focus on what she is experiencing by calling her attention to the smells and sounds as well as the fascinating sights.

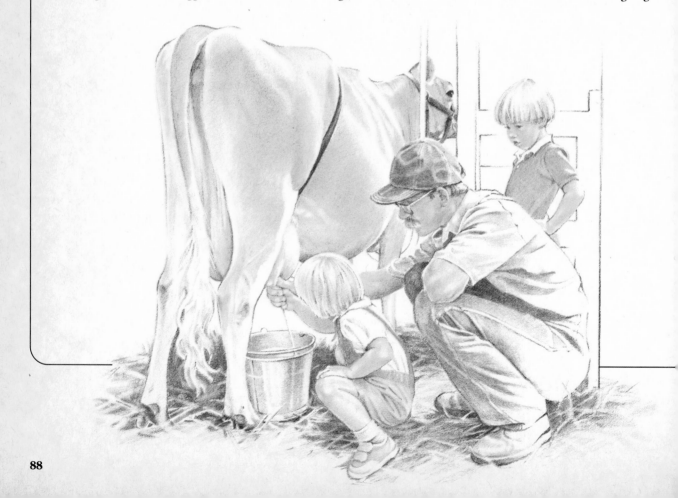

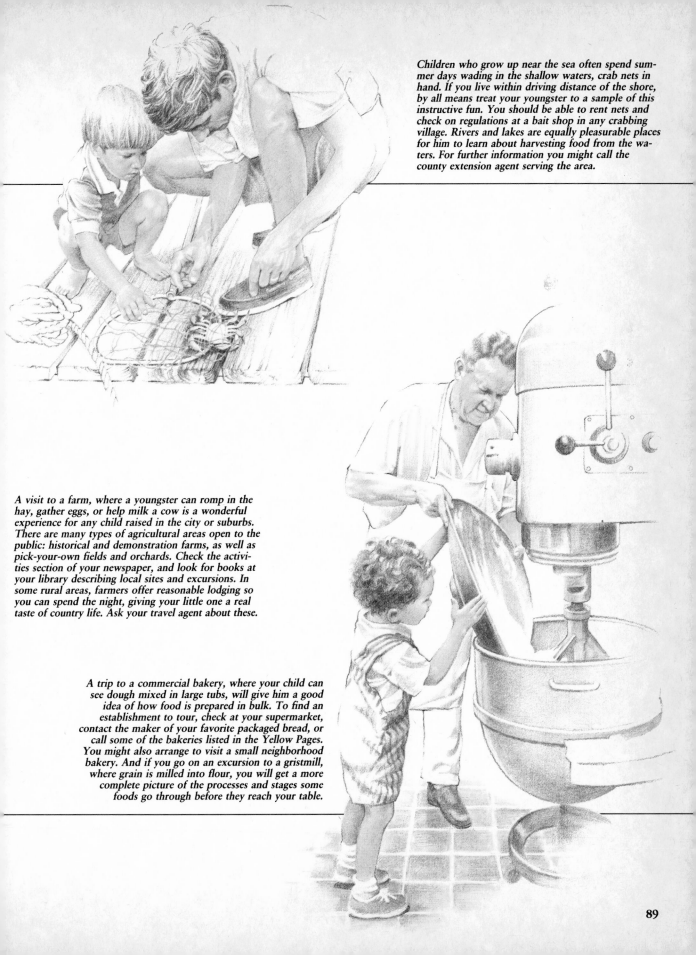

Children who grow up near the sea often spend summer days wading in the shallow waters, crab nets in hand. If you live within driving distance of the shore, by all means treat your youngster to a sample of this instructive fun. You should be able to rent nets and check on regulations at a bait shop in any crabbing village. Rivers and lakes are equally pleasurable places for him to learn about harvesting food from the waters. For further information you might call the county extension agent serving the area.

A visit to a farm, where a youngster can romp in the hay, gather eggs, or help milk a cow is a wonderful experience for any child raised in the city or suburbs. There are many types of agricultural areas open to the public: historical and demonstration farms, as well as pick-your-own fields and orchards. Check the activities section of your newspaper, and look for books at your library describing local sites and excursions. In some rural areas, farmers offer reasonable lodging so you can spend the night, giving your little one a real taste of country life. Ask your travel agent about these.

A trip to a commercial bakery, where your child can see dough mixed in large tubs, will give him a good idea of how food is prepared in bulk. To find an establishment to tour, check at your supermarket, contact the maker of your favorite packaged bread, or call some of the bakeries listed in the Yellow Pages. You might also arrange to visit a small neighborhood bakery. And if you go on an excursion to a gristmill, where grain is milled into flour, you will get a more complete picture of the processes and stages some foods go through before they reach your table.

Growing Things at Home

The idea that a sturdy vine will grow from a sweet potato and a plant sprout from a tiny radish seed will amaze your youngster. As she observes the changes day to day, she will gain firsthand knowledge of the plant life cycle.

A few rules ensure success. Planting may be done in pots indoors and the pots moved outside when the weather warms. Be sure that each container has one large or several small drainage holes in the bottom; and place pebbles or broken bits of a flower pot in the bottom for drainage. Fill each container with potting soil and follow the directions on the seed packets. Before the seeds sprout, cover the pot with plastic wrap and keep it in a warm place, away from direct light. Once the seedlings emerge, remove the plastic and place the plant by a sunny window. Green peppers, peas, beans, and miniature carrots are easy to grow, and green onions are fun because the hollow leaves can be used as straws in tomato juice.

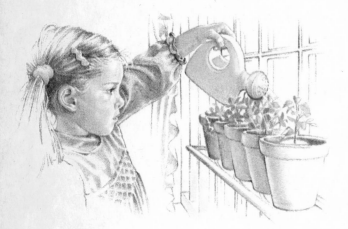

If you have a window that gets sun for most of the day, you might want to start an indoor herb garden with your child. Basil, dill, oregano, sage, and thyme sprout readily. A milk carton with one long side cut away makes a good window box, or you can grow the herbs in individual pots. When the plants have leafed out, let your child cut some sprigs and add the savory clippings to your dishes.

Cherry tomatoes seem to be particularly satisfying for children to grow, perhaps because the youngsters identify with the fruits' diminutive size. Following the instructions on the packet, sow seeds indoors in early spring; as the seedlings sprout and develop second leaves, pull out all but the strongest one. When the plant is about four inches high and the danger of frost is past, transplant it to a sunny garden plot or to a larger flowerpot on a sunny terrace.

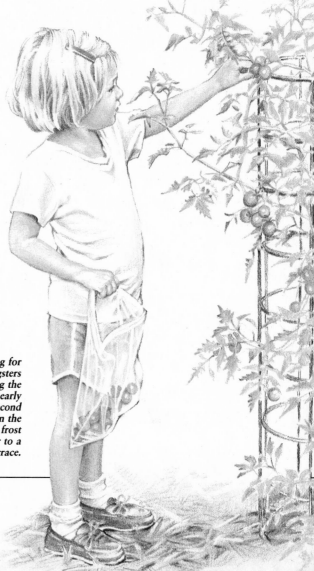

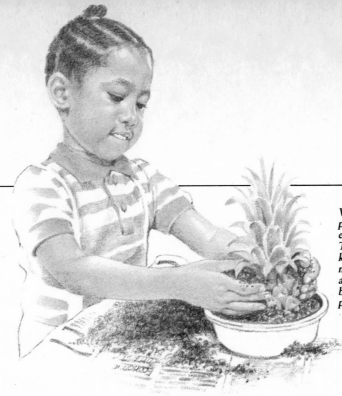

With patience, your youngster can coax the top of a pineapple into producing a small fruit. Let the cut edge, with one inch of flesh attached, dry for a day. Then plant the top in a flowerpot. Water it daily and keep it in a sunny place. Once it has begun to grow new leaves, put the pot in a plastic bag with a ripe apple (the apple stimulates bud formation), seal the bag, and store it in darkness until a central shoot appears. From this will sprout a pineapple.

The way egg whites fluff up when beaten is one of the more dramatic phenomena in the culinary world. To ensure perfect results, follow a meringue recipe in one of your cookbooks. Give your child a bowl, a hand beater, and egg whites brought to room temperature. While your little cook beats, you can gradually add sugar and then some vanilla. The fluff can then be baked into tasty cookies. When beating the whites, the cookie maker may be most comfortable on the floor, where he can get a good grip on both bowl and beater.

Experiments in the Kitchen

Although it is easier to pull a pizza from the freezer, or open a jar of applesauce than to make either, there is something gratifying about preparing a dish from scratch. A rainy weekend provides the perfect opportunity for you and your child to indulge in a culinary fest with some of his favorite foods. The four described above and on the next page are ones your child can either create himself or help prepare. Before you begin, see the safety instructions on page 94.

As he beats, kneads, churns, and sifts, he will learn that preparing food takes time, patience, and a bit of elbow grease. And he will also discover the pleasure of seeing something take shape in direct response to his various actions. Talk about textures and the delicious aromas as you cook and do not discourage an occasional tasting of the dish in progress.

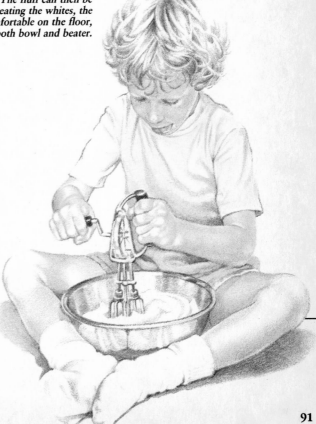

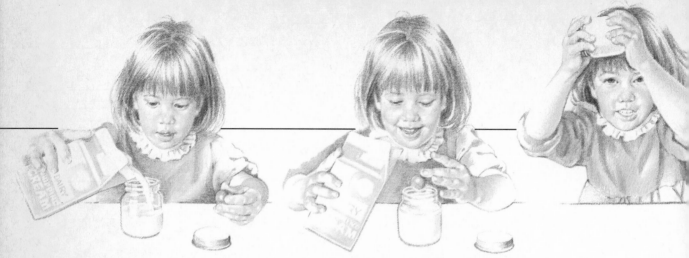

Equipped with chilled heavy cream, a marble, and a jar, your youngster can churn her own butter in about fifteen minutes. Have her partially fill a small jar with the cream. Next, have her drop in a clean marble, cover the jar, and shake it vigorously. Those little arms will tire soon. You will want to take turns shaking. As the butter forms, the sound of the marble rat- tling will cease. Pour out the remaining liquid, or but- termilk, pressing the butter with a wooden spoon to compact it. Save the buttermilk to drink, if you like, or use it for pancakes. Chill a bit of the butter, then spread it on bread or crackers; everything will taste that much better if the bread is homemade and just out of the oven.

Applesauce is a perfect follow-up activity after a trip to an orchard. Your child will have a chance to see how a food goes from its source to his tummy. Get out your favorite recipe. You probably ought to take charge of peeling, slicing, and cooking the apples; when the apples have cooled, your helper can process them through a food mill or press their pulp through a sieve with the back of a wooden spoon. If you like, you can try something new and cook the sauce with grated orange peel, then spice it afterward with the usual nutmeg and cinnamon. Explain that one of the rewards of making foods at home is that you can ad- just flavors to suit yourself.

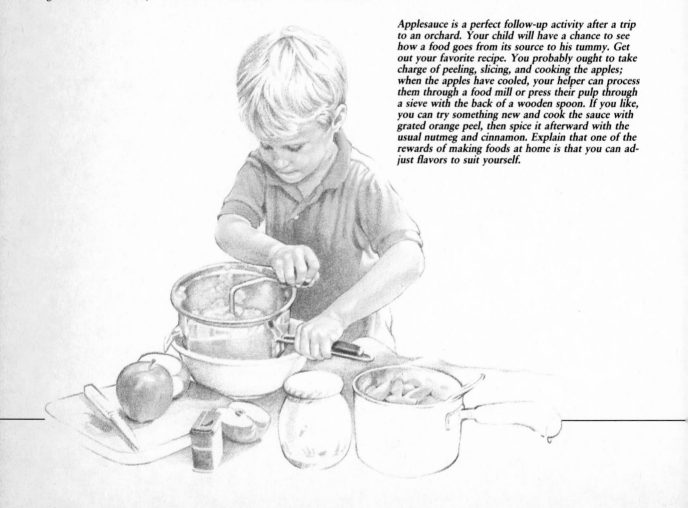

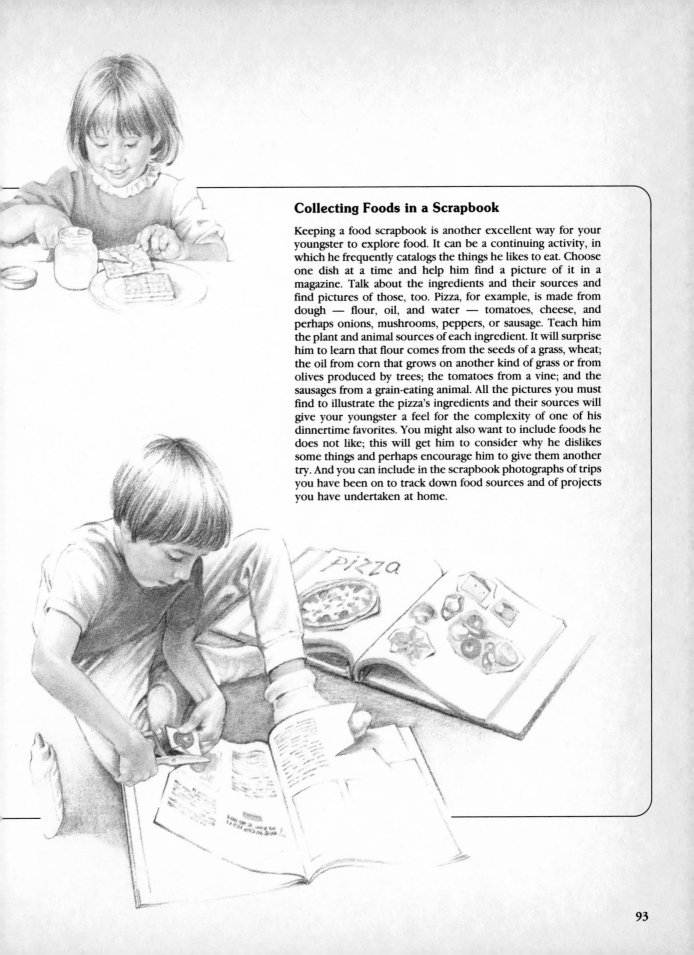

Collecting Foods in a Scrapbook

Keeping a food scrapbook is another excellent way for your youngster to explore food. It can be a continuing activity, in which he frequently catalogs the things he likes to eat. Choose one dish at a time and help him find a picture of it in a magazine. Talk about the ingredients and their sources and find pictures of those, too. Pizza, for example, is made from dough — flour, oil, and water — tomatoes, cheese, and perhaps onions, mushrooms, peppers, or sausage. Teach him the plant and animal sources of each ingredient. It will surprise him to learn that flour comes from the seeds of a grass, wheat; the oil from corn that grows on another kind of grass or from olives produced by trees; the tomatoes from a vine; and the sausages from a grain-eating animal. All the pictures you must find to illustrate the pizza's ingredients and their sources will give your youngster a feel for the complexity of one of his dinnertime favorites. You might also want to include foods he does not like; this will get him to consider why he dislikes some things and perhaps encourage him to give them another try. And you can include in the scrapbook photographs of trips you have been on to track down food sources and of projects you have undertaken at home.

Getting Ready to Cook

Most children are ready for their first simple culinary adventures at around the age of two. All it takes is a little forethought on your part. Your toddler may enjoy patting a hamburger between two pudgy palms or delight in cutting out cookies with interestingly shaped plastic forms. In another year or so, she will be able to perform such tasks as washing vegetables, shelling peas, and pouring out ingredients that have already been measured. By four or five, she may be quite skillful and feeling very useful and adult, cracking eggs, grating cheese, measuring ingredients, and mixing batters on her own.

Whether your youngster is six or two, you will want to keep a few guidelines in mind when you and she cook together. First, as with most activities, make sure that your little one is well rested and in good spirits; a tired or irritable child will not enjoy learning something new or even helping with familiar rituals. If she is hungry, give her a light snack so she will not be distracted by a growly stomach. For your part, be prepared for some messiness. And make certain that you have plenty of time to devote to the venture; when time is short, it is better to wait for another day than to risk becoming impatient with your child's naturally slower pace. After all, you are initiating the activity and inviting her to join you. In any case, by choosing a simple recipe, you are far less likely to feel pressured. And if you have to complete the preparations if your young cook's attention wanders, you will not be unnecessarily inconvenienced.

Before getting started, you should spend fifteen minutes or so setting the scene and preparing the kitchen — clearing counters and arranging utensils and ingredients. Having everything handy allows you to concentrate on the project with your child, rather than rummaging in cabinets for one item after another. Take time to talk with her about what you two will do; show her the ingredients and let her smell and feel them.

Your small helper will need plenty of space in which to work, since she is likely to be a bit awkward until she gets the hang of things. You might want to have a special low table just for her use; but if there is no room in your kitchen, have her stand on a sturdy wooden chair while she is working at the counter.

You will want to get your young cook ready, as well. If she is wearing long sleeves, roll them up, so they will not get in the foods. Tie back long hair. And teach her to wash her hands anytime she is going to be working in the kitchen. While a few germs may not harm anything, now is a good time for her to learn the importance of cleanliness when handling food.

Finally, give careful thought to safety in the kitchen. Be there to help and supervise from start to finish. Explain that the stove is likely to be hot when you are preparing food, and that it will burn her if she touches it. Keep all pans on the stove with the handles turned inward and never allow your child near the stove when you are cooking with hot oil. Show her that knives are sharp by slicing vegetables — always cutting away from your body. Gradually teach her to use knives properly, starting with a relatively safe serrated plastic knife and graduating over time to a regular serrated knife with a blunt end.

Show her how electrical appliances work and emphasize that they are to be turned on only when an adult says so. There is no need for long lectures on these potential hazards, however; matter-of-fact explanations and an occasional reminder should be sufficient. In all likelihood, your child will learn the most about safety in the kitchen by watching the way you work. So be on your mettle to practice good habits.

First Tasks

Many basic culinary tasks involve little or no equipment. Cracking eggs, snapping beans, and pressing out meat patties — pictured below — require only clean hands and a bowl or plate to hold the food. Other jobs, such as scrubbing vegetables and wrapping potatoes in foil for baking, are more a matter of using hands skillfully than of manipulating utensils. For this reason, many young children find such things easier to master and more enjoyable than those tasks that do require special equipment. They also appeal because youngsters just naturally like to get their hands into food. Nevertheless, some of these jobs are harder than others; cracking eggs, for instance, takes a fair amount of eye-hand coordination — and considerable practice.

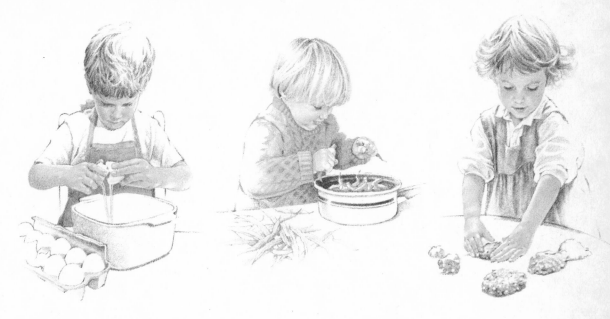

Measuring

By the time your youngster is ready to measure ingredients, she will be perfectly familiar with measuring cups and spoons, having already played with them. Start your little one off with dry ingredients, since, as the picture shows, she need only learn to sweep a spatula—or even a finger—across the top of the spoon to level the contents. Pouring liquids to a particular line on a cup is more difficult. Putting a piece of tape on the target mark — as illustrated below — will show your youngster at what point to stop pouring.

Using Utensils

Kitchen appliances are fascinating to your budding cook, who will soon discover that with their help she can do all kinds of interesting things with foods. Hand-operated tools, such as the juicer below, are ideal, since your youngster can manage them on her own. When you set your child up with a piece of kitchen equipment, make sure that she is situated high enough to be able to use it properly; do not however, have her stand on a stool, which may wobble. With the juicer, she should be able to press down hard on the oranges and twist from her elbow rather than her wrist.

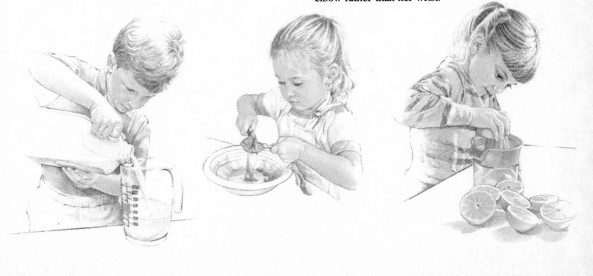

Starting Simple

There are any number of ways to combine ingredients, using everything from your hands to a high-powered food processor. In general, children do best with simple tools and relate more readily to jobs that bring them close to the food. Stirring batter with a wooden spoon, beating eggs with a whisk, mixing flour, baking powder, and salt with a sifter, and kneading meat loaf by hand are among the most satisfying of such endeavors. It is a good idea to have the ingredients measured out beforehand; and bowls should be flat-bottomed and sturdy. When an electrical appliance is the best utensil for the job, the activity is really suitable only for an older child and even then, an adult should of course supervise closely. Your preschooler can help out by pouring ingredients into the pitcher or bowl and, perhaps, pressing the on-off button while you stand nearby.

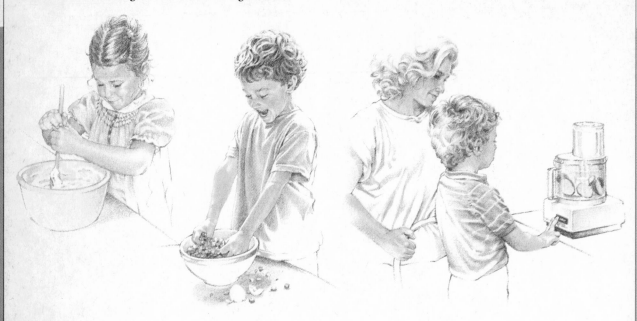

Handling Knives and Sharp Instruments

Chopping, slicing, and peeling are basic to the preparation of many dishes, but tasks such as these, which entail the use of sharp utensils, should be taught to your youngster gradually. When she is four years of age or mature enough to handle it, have her use a knife with a rounded tip and a serrated edge. With it she can slice cheese and softer vegetables such as large mushrooms, peppers, and cucumbers. A parer is an appropriate cutting tool for a slightly older child, who has the coordination to peel vegetables with the necessary sweeping motion away from his body and can understand that the inner edges are sharp. A grater is another suitable tool for a preschooler; just caution her not to grate all the way to the end of the item or she will scrape her fingers.

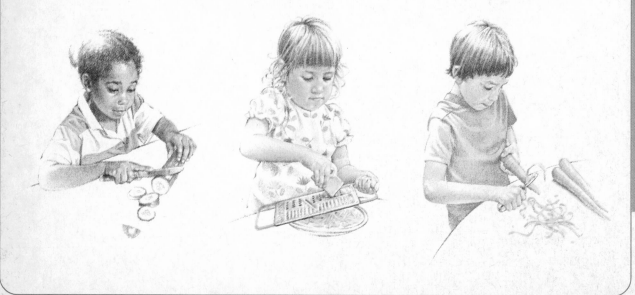

Baking

Baking is a perfect activity to let your child help you with since many of the associated tasks are safe for little fingers. Greasing pans and cookie sheets, punching down dough or rolling it flat with a rolling pin, cutting out cookies, and spooning batter into muffin tins all take place away from the stove and do not require the use of sharp utensils or electrical appliances. Another reason your youngster may enjoy playing baker is that the results are so wonderfully satisfying: At the end, the cold and gooey stuff goes into the oven and minutes later, out it comes, firm and warmly golden — and, of course, a delight to her and the rest of the family.

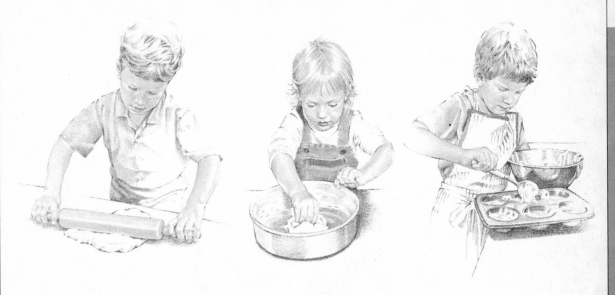

Cooking on a Burner

By about the age of five, many children are mature enough to begin to cook on top of the stove — with adult supervision, naturally. Choose simple dishes that require only a few minutes' actual cooking time and avoid anything that demands hot oil. Scrambled eggs, which cook best over low heat, are a good starting point; so are pancakes — fast-cooking and fun to flip and watch bubble. Be sure your child uses potholders when holding hot items — and stay near her while she works.

Cleaning Up

If you treat cleaning up as a part of the kitchen experience, your youngster will probably accept it readily and enjoy washing dishes. The soapy water is fun and he will feel grown-up in the bargain. When you are cooking, teach your child to wipe or sweep up spills as they happen, so someone does not slip. Encourage cooperation by asking him to hold the dustpan for you. But remember that a little mess is the price of creativity and do not fuss if he sprinkles flour on the floor or winds up with batter all over his shirt.

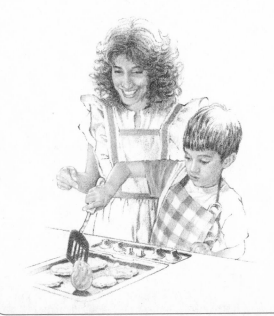

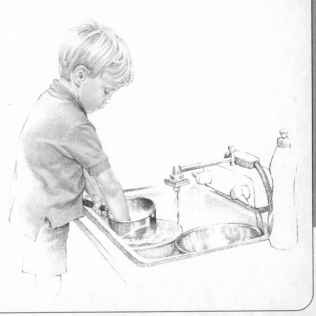

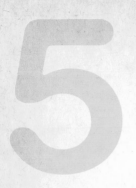

Practical Cooking for Hungry Youngsters

Being a good cook means being a good shopper —
buying the freshest and the best and preparing your
purchases in ways that will preserve as much of their
inherent goodness as possible. The effort this involves
is slight, and it pays off in benefits not only for your
child but also for the whole family.

In the pages that follow, you will find tips for buying
and storing food, as well as information on which
cooking methods are soundest from a nutritional point
of view. For mothers who want to go to the extra
trouble, there is a section on making baby foods at
home, a task rendered easier today by the food
processor. And finally, to whet your young one's
appetite, a minicookbook offers more than thirty
recipes suitable not just for the under-six set, but for
the rest of the family as well. Most contain steps your
budding cook can help you with, as the child in the
photograph at right is doing. Besides being fun to
prepare, these recipes will enlarge his interest in food
as he comes to understand more about the cooking
process itself, with all its magical transformations,
wonderful aromas, and delicious end products.

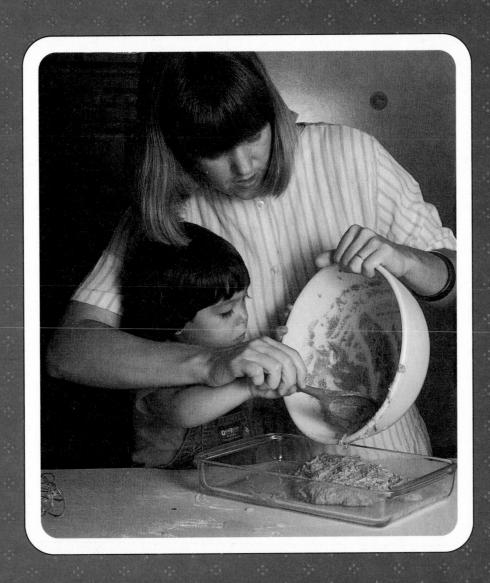

Planning and Preparing Wholesome Meals

Seeing that your youngster gets a balanced diet means shopping for good, fresh food, handling it properly when you get it home, and preparing it in such a way that as much as possible of its nutrient value is preserved.

Looking for the best
To obtain both quality and value, tailor your menu and your shopping list to whatever local fruits and vegetables are in season in your area. Local produce usually is reasonably priced, so you can afford to buy the best quality. Try to buy small quantities two or three times a week, so that you can use the fruits and vegetables when they are still fresh.

Although specific shopping tips vary for each fruit or vegetable, there are a few general rules to follow. Avoid pre-wrapped packages, which may hide bruises and flaws. Moderately sized, young, brightly-colored produce is best; large, overgrown specimens are tougher and less flavorful. Tasty citrus fruit can be chosen by weight rather than size, since a sweet, juicy fruit is denser and heavier than a dry, pulpy one.

Most fruit is best bought nearly ripe, neither green nor soft. Some fruits, such as papayas, bananas, and pears, can be purchased green and ripened at home. Apples are best bought and eaten when firm and crisp.

Drawbacks of processed foods
Processed products present both choices and problems. For nutritional value, frozen foods rank second to good, fresh ones, because the prefreeze peeling and parboiling they require leach away some vitamins and minerals. Canned foods rank third in flavor and nutrition, because heating during the canning process affects the heat-sensitive vitamins and because most canned food contains excess sugar or salt.

Processing, particularly in the manufacture of packaged foods, involves the addition of various substances, either to enhance the foods' nutritive value or to extend their shelf life. Products containing preservatives and stabilizers cannot be avoided in this age of convenience, but you will wish to choose the foods lowest in these additives by checking labels.

Selecting meat, poultry, and fish
Most parents want their children to eat animal protein and seek the best meat when shopping. But the well-marbled piece of beef, so long upheld as the paragon of taste and juiciness, is no longer preferred by nutritionists. Lean cuts are better for health, and you can render them even more healthful by removing any visible fat (*box, opposite*). The white meat of chicken and turkey is another lean source of protein, if its skin is removed.

A Cook's Primer of Beef

To lower the fat in your child's diet, pay close attention to the kind of meat you buy. Keep in mind that labeling terms vary from market to market; "lean," for example, may not be as lean as you think. The U.S. Department of Agriculture grades include Prime, Choice, and Select. Prime and Choice are quite tender and flavorful, but high in fat; Select has less fat. When pur-chasing ground beef for hamburgers or casseroles, consider buying whole cuts, such as top and bottom round, eye round, and sirloin tip, trimming any visible fat, and grinding the meat at home. When trimmed, such cuts have a maximum of 37 percent of their calories in fat, as opposed to regular, lean, and extra lean ground beef, which have much higher percentages (*below*).

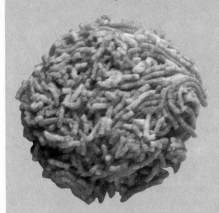
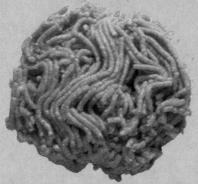
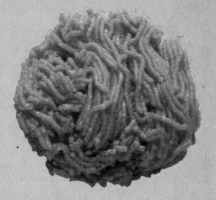

Regular ground beef, less red than the leaner examples because of its high fat content, still has about 65 percent of its calories in fat even after broiling.

Lean ground beef like this, when cooked, has 61 percent of its calories in fat.

Extra lean ground beef, typically bright red, has about 58 percent of its calories from fat. It often must be custom-ground.

Storing food for health

Proper storage helps preserve the nutrients in food. Fresh food loses flavor and vitamins in three ways, all of them preventable. Warm temperatures accelerate enzymatic breakdown and bacterial growth, effects that are slowed by refrigeration and freezer storage. Light also hastens deterioration. And air tends to dehydrate fresh foods and leach away nutrients.

Before refrigerating fruit, make certain that it is ripe. If it is not ready to eat when you buy it, keep it at room temperature (ideally between 65° F. and 80° F.) away from direct sunlight. To speed the process, place the fruit first in a paper bag. Then, when it has ripened, refrigerate it. Most vegetables should be wrapped in plastic and stored in the hydrator or crisper, usually the bottom drawer, where the humidity reduces moisture loss; exceptions include white potatoes, sweet potatoes, winter squash, and onions, which can be stored in any cool, dark, dry location. To minimize moisture loss, remove the leafy tops from beets, carrots, and similar roots before refrigerating them. For the same reason leave on peels and pods, which seal in not only moisture, but vitamins and minerals too.

Proper refrigeration is particularly important for protein-rich foods — meat, poultry, fish, dairy products, and eggs — and for dishes made with them, as well as for cooked starches, such as potatoes and rice. Because such foods are moist, they can provide bacteria with a rich environment in which to grow.

To minimize these foods' exposure to temperatures between

40° F. and 140° F., which encourage bacteria to proliferate, refrigerate or freeze them immediately after shopping. Put meat in your refrigerator's meat keeper, the coldest compartment, where temperatures range between 32° F. and 40° F. Tightly-wrapped ground meat can be kept for about two days; whole cuts, loosely wrapped so that air will dry the surface enough to keep it from being a host to bacteria, may be kept three or four days. When in doubt, read butcher labels; the date beyond which the meat may no longer be held should be written there (*box, right*). Store milk, cheese, and dairy products close to the refrigerator's coldest part. You can keep closed jars, condiments, and grains stored in tight containers on the middle shelves, where the temperature is about 40° F., on the door shelves, or on the bottom shelf, the warmest area.

Cook food soon after removing it from the refrigerator to deter growth of bacteria or loss of nutrients. Promptly refrigerate any leftovers. Never allow cooked food to cool gradually at room temperature; if it is too hot to put immediately in the refrigerator, transfer it whenever possible to a number of smaller containers so that it can cool more quickly. And be particularly careful to chill protein-rich picnic foods, such as chicken and potato salad and barbecued chicken and hamburgers; left outdoors in summer, these can become food-poisoning hazards within an hour or two.

You can freeze both raw and cooked foods and they will hold their nutritional value well at temperatures below 0° F. Before freezing an item, seal it in airtight wrappings or containers to prevent moisture and nutrient losses. Thaw the frozen food in the refrigerator, not at room temperature. Then be sure to use the thawed food within a day or two. Do not refreeze precooked foods. Keep in mind that while freezing has its advantages, precooked food will lose additional vitamins and flavor in the reheating process.

Keeping things clean

When preparing food, cleanliness is the rule. The most important precaution against contamination is good old-fashioned handwashing. Wash your hands before you start cooking and again after each interruption — after reading, picking up your child, or changing his diapers. And wash your hands as well after handling raw meat, fish, or poultry, which often harbor bacteria. Utensils, particularly those used to cut up poultry and fish, should be cleaned with soap and hot water, as should countertops and cutting boards, where bacteria from the food can easily multiply.

Decoding Freshness Labels

From a shopper's viewpoint, the dates on food labels leave much to be desired. There is no nationwide standard, merely a crazy quilt of state laws. Nor do manufacturers always explain the meaning of their dated labels. For aid in deciphering a cryptic dating system, ask your grocer. If he cannot tell you, telephone the manufacturer. Here, to help you, is a key to basic terms:

Sell by. Often called a pull date, this is the last date a store should sell a product, allowing a reasonable period for home storage and use.

Best if used by. Commonly used on meat and cheese, this reflects the time limit for optimum freshness, after which taste and nutrient value may suffer although the product is not necessarily dangerous to eat.

Expiration date. Often seen on baby food, milk, and yeast, this is the last day the item should be used. Be sure to discard foods after their expiration date.

Pack date. Used on some frozen and canned goods, pack date stands for the day on which a product was manufactured. It is useful only if you know the product's shelf life. For safety and good nutrition, frozen food generally should be used within four months, canned goods within a year.

Preserving nutrients Although cooking inevitably diminishes a food's nutrient content somewhat, you can minimize loss with a good choice of cooking method. In addition to destroying heat-sensitive vitamins, cooking removes some nutrients through evaporation and literally throws other nutrients away with the cooking liquid. Nutrient losses occur less with methods that call for little or no water, such as microwaving, steaming, pressure-cooking, and stir-frying. In addition to being fast — which means that the food's exposure to heat is fairly brief — microwaving ensures that vegetables will retain much of their coloration and be more appetizing. Braises, soups, and stews minimize nutrient loss by capturing minerals and vitamins in the cooking liquid; boiling, broiling, and frying waste nutrients unless the juices or liquids are incorporated into sauces or in soup. If the juices from braised and broiled meat are used this way, the fat should be removed. This can be accomplished by letting liquid cool so that the fat rises to the surface and can be skimmed off, or by chilling the juices, then removing the congealed fat on top.

A few words to the wise Not only can the method of cooking you choose have an effect on the nutrient value of the food, but it can also determine the outcome, especially as to tenderness and flavor. Cooked slowly over medium heat, perhaps with tomatoes (whose acid acts as a tenderizing agent), then sliced thin, lean meats lose their toughness. Like red meat, poultry also benefits from slow cooking with liquid, which helps keep in the juices and minimize shrinkage. By contrast, protein-rich fish should be cooked quickly; too much exposure to heat will leave it dried out and deprived of much of its flavor.

Tending to vegetables Vegetables, a mainstay of your child's diet, should be washed briefly in cold water just before cooking and immediately cut up. Exposing them to light or air for a long period or leaving them to soak will lead to a loss of nutrients. Consider the value of not peeling them; vegetable skins are rich in minerals, vitamins, and fiber. Indeed, carrots, potatoes, and the like are better eaten unpeeled; vegetables that must be peeled, such as turnips, beets, and winter squash, might be cooked in their skins and peeled afterward. Remember that all vegetables are best served freshly cooked, but if you have leftovers, do not reheat them, for this will reduce nutrients even more. Instead, serve them cold, with a vinaigrette dressing or in a salad. Your child will love them. ❖

Making Baby Food at Home

Commercial baby food today is convenient and wholesome, without the extra sugar and salt that earned it a negative reputation a few years ago. But many parents prefer to make their own purees and use these as a mainstay of their young one's diet or as a supplement to jarred foods.

Although homemade purees take more time to prepare than simply opening and warming a jar, they have several virtues. They are about half the cost of commercial baby food. They provide excellent nutrition, free of the stabilizers and starch fillers sometimes used in the store-bought product. They give you the chance to make baby food from components of almost any family meal. And for convenience, they can be made in large batches, then frozen in individual portions.

Your baby needs pureed foods for about three months or so only, beginning around six months, when you can start her on pureed fruits and vegetables as well as poultry, veal, and beef. You will want, of course, to introduce one new food at a time, pausing three days between foods to see whether the baby shows any intolerance to the item just tried. By nine months, she can move on to such foods as raw, ripe bananas, pears, and peaches, cottage cheese, and mashed, well-cooked vegetables, as well as mashed lamb and liver that have been thinned with a little broth or juices. At twelve months she can eat chopped, bite-size pieces of table food.

Your decision as to whether you should go ahead and make your own baby food will probably depend on time and cost constraints. Preparing baby food requires no special equipment, although having a food processor can be a great time-saver. Steaming, an excellent way to cook vegetables for maximum nutrition, requires only a folding basket that fits inside a pot with a tight-fitting lid. If you do not have a food processor, you can make purees with a hand-cranked food mill, an electric blender, or an inexpensive, portable baby-food grinder.

When selecting ingredients, be sure to use fresh, high-quality groceries, not your leftovers, which

After filling an ice-cube tray with pureed carrots, this mother will freeze the tray. Later, she will transfer the frozen cubes to a plastic freezer bag for storage.

lose nutrients when they are reheated. Fruit should be very ripe. Commercial frozen vegetables can be used provided that they contain no added sugar or salt. Fresh or frozen lean meat can also be used, but stay away from corned, smoked, salt- and sugar-cured meats, or canned ones, which contain far more sodium than your child needs.

A step-by-step guide

Seed and core fruits and vegetables. For meat and poultry, trim away all visible fat and remove any chicken or turkey skin. Cut up or chop the food into pieces that are one or two inches long. Do not add salt or sugar.

You will probably want to steam or microwave raw vegetables and fruits in order to conserve their nutrients. Allow vegetables to cook until they are tender but not limp or discolored. If you do not wish to steam or microwave them, you can boil them rapidly in a small amount of water and use a bit of the cooking liquid to thin the puree. Fruit can also be poached until tender (usually for 15 to 30 minutes) in an inch or two of simmering water. Meat should be simmered on medium heat until very tender — about 45 minutes for veal or chicken, approximately 90 minutes for beef. Vegetables such as celery, carrots, and potatoes can be added 35 minutes before the meat has finished cooking; this will prevent them from overcooking and surrendering too many of their nutrients. Save the juices so that you can add them to the puree when you grind up the meat and vegetables.

Let the food cool slightly. Using one-cup batches for meats and two-cup batches for vegetables and fruits, puree the cooked food until all lumps disappear. Add cooking liquid as needed to achieve a smooth, thick consistency.

Immediately pour the warm puree into plastic ice-cube trays, or into clean baby-food jars to a level about one inch from the rim. Spread wax paper over the trays and loosely cap the jars and place them in the freezer immediately (after the jars' contents begin to congeal, tighten the lids). Let the cubes freeze for at least eight hours, then tip them out of the trays into a plastic freezer bag and seal it. Frozen purees will keep safely for at least a month.

To serve your homemade frozen purees, take one or two cubes or a jar from the freezer and allow them to thaw in a double boiler, or in the refrigerator. In the case of the jar, loosen the cap. If you microwave the jar, be sure to remove the cap and replace it with plastic wrap that has been pierced to prevent steam buildup. ⋰

Foods to Be Wary Of

Here is a list of foods and beverages that may cause choking, trigger sensitivity reactions, or promote bad eating habits in children younger than two years and a shorter list of foods that may be fine for children over one but dangerous to younger children.

Under 2 Years

- Caffeinated beverages
- Corn
- Fried or fatty food
- Fruit with seeds
- Fruit, dried
- Grapes, whole
- Hot dogs
- Nuts, especially peanuts
- Olives
- Peanut butter
- Popcorn
- Salty food
- Spicy food
- Sugary foods and drinks
- Vegetables, raw— such as carrot and celery sticks, green beans and cauliflower

Under 1 Year

- Chocolate
- Berries, fresh
- Egg whites
- Fruit, citrus
- Honey
- Luncheon meats
- Raisins

Recipes with Child Appeal

The thirty-four recipes that follow were created especially for this volume using ingredients low in sodium, high in fiber, and rich in such important nutrients as vitamins A and C, calcium, and iron. The recipes have also been designed with simplicity in mind; many of the steps — indicated by red bullets in each recipe — can be performed by your young child, providing you with an opportunity to involve him in the cooking process. This will be one factor in enticing your little one to try new foods; so will a dish that is pleasing to the eye and displayed on a brightly colored plate or arranged to make the most of a food's natural color and texture.

In preparing any of the recipes containing margarine, butter, or oil, take into account the fat content of the rest of the day's menu to be certain that no more than 35 percent of your child's calories will be from fat, the top limit set by the National Academy of Sciences. Depending on your child's age, you will want to modify the serving portions to reflect his appetite.

Breakfasts

Cornmeal-Blueberry Pancakes

Makes 8 large pancakes

> 1 cup all-purpose flour
> ½ cup yellow cornmeal
> 3 tbsp. sugar
> 1½ tsp. baking powder
> 2 eggs
> 3 tbsp. vegetable oil
> 1 cup buttermilk or 1 cup plain low-fat yogurt
> 1 cup fresh or frozen unsweetened blueberries

- Sift the flour, cornmeal, sugar, and baking powder together.
- In a mixing bowl, whisk together the eggs, oil, and buttermilk or yogurt.
- Add the dry ingredients to the egg mixture and stir just until the flour is blended in; do not overmix.
- Stir in the blueberries.
- Heat a large nonstick or heavy-bottomed skillet over medium heat. If the pan does not have a nonstick coating, add 2 teaspoons of vegetable oil. The pan is hot enough when a few drops of water sprinkled onto the surface skitter about and evaporate

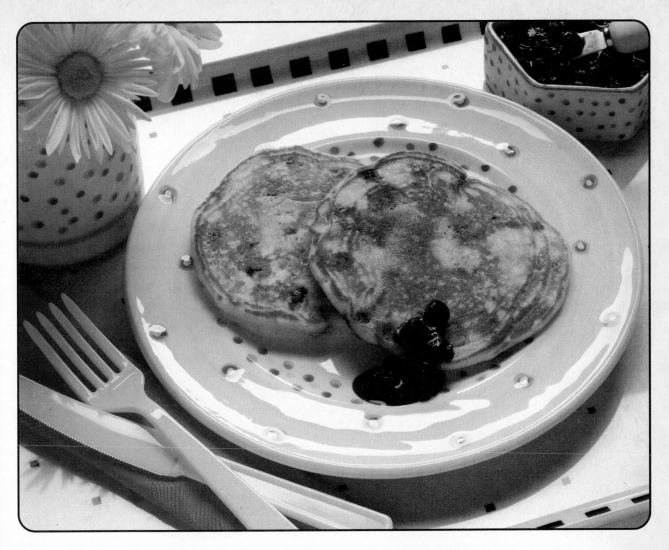

almost instantly. Spoon about ⅓ cup of the batter into the skillet and spread it to make a pancake about 4 inches across. Cook the pancake on the first side until bubbles begin to form and the underside is well browned; turn the pancake over and cook the other side until it too is brown. Repeat with the remaining batter. To keep them hot, the pancakes can be placed in a 200° F. oven until the last one is ready. Serve the pancakes hot, with blueberry-orange syrup *(recipe below)*, if you like.

Blueberry-Orange Syrup

Makes 1½ cups

1½ cup fresh or frozen unsweetened blueberries
¼ cup orange-juice concentrate

- Put the blueberries into a small saucepan and stir in the orange-juice concentrate.
- Bring the mixture to a simmer over low heat and cook the syrup, stirring frequently, until heated through. Serve warm.

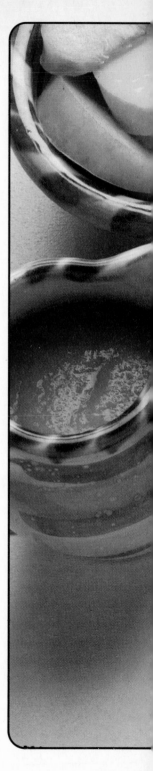

Whole-Wheat Waffles

Makes 4 double waffles

¾ cup whole-wheat flour
¾ cup all-purpose flour
4 tsp. baking powder
2 tbsp. sugar
2 eggs
1 cup low-fat or skim milk
2 tbsp. vegetable oil

- Preheat a waffle iron to medium high. If you are not using a nonstick waffle iron, lightly oil the inside surfaces of the iron.
- Sift the flours, baking powder, and sugar together.
- With a mixer or whisk blend the eggs, milk, and oil together.
- Add the flour mixture and stir just until the flour is blended in; do not overmix.
- Spread one-fourth of the batter on the waffle iron, close the lid, and bake the waffle until it is brown and comes away easily from the waffle iron—about five minutes. If you want to have all of the waffles ready at the same time, keep the cooked waffles warm in a 200° F. oven while you bake the others. Serve the waffles hot, with peach-maple waffle syrup *(recipe below),* if you like.

Variations

Peach-Pecan Waffles: Prepare as above, but after adding the flour, gently stir in ½ cup chopped fresh peaches or frozen, unsweetened peaches and ½ cup chopped pecans.

Apple Waffles: Prepare as above, but after adding the flour, add ½ cup chopped fresh apples or canned, unsweetened apple to the batter, stirring gently.

Peach-Maple Waffle Syrup

This syrup is delicious whether it is made with fresh, frozen, or canned peaches. If you are using canned peaches, use the kind that are packed in juice rather than in syrup.

Makes about 2 cups

1¾ cups chopped peaches
⅓ cup maple syrup

- Puree the peaches in a food processor or a blender and transfer the puree to a small saucepan.
- Stir in the maple syrup.
- Bring the mixture to a simmer over low heat, partially cover the pan, and cook the syrup for five minutes, stirring several times. Serve warm or at room temperature.

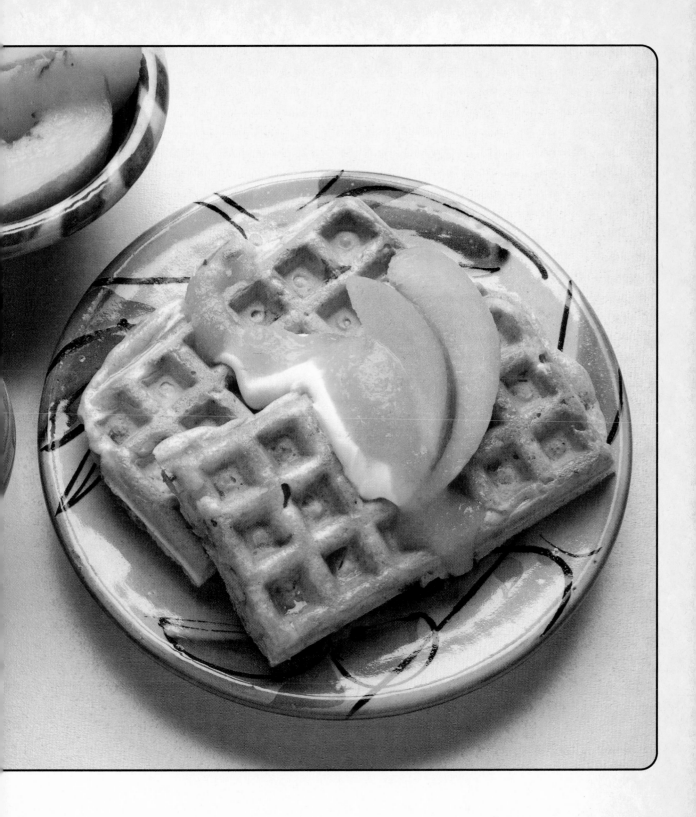

Popover Pancake

The applesauce accompanying this pancake may be warmed, if you like.

Serves 4

> 3 eggs
> ¼ cup all-purpose flour
> ¼ cup whole wheat flour
> ½ cup low-fat or skim milk
> 2 tbsp. vegetable oil
> 2 tbsp. margarine or butter
> 2 tbsp. confectioners' sugar
> 1 lemon, cut into four wedges
> 1 cup applesauce

- Preheat the oven to 425° F.
- In a bowl beat the eggs, flours, and milk together until ingredients are blended.
- Heat the oil and the margarine or butter in a heavy 10-inch ovenproof skillet set over medium heat. When the margarine or butter begins to foam, pour in the batter all at once.
- Cook the pancake on top of the stove until it begins to firm up— about two minutes. Loosen the edges of the pancake with a spatula, then slip the spatula under the center of the pancake and quickly flip the pancake over. (The batter will still be loose; do not worry if the pancake looks messy.
- Transfer the skillet to the oven and bake the pancake until it is puffed and brown all over — about 15 minutes.
- Sprinkle the pancake with the confectioners' sugar, cut it into four pieces, and serve each slice with a wedge of lemon, which can be squeezed over the pancake. Serve the slices with applesauce.

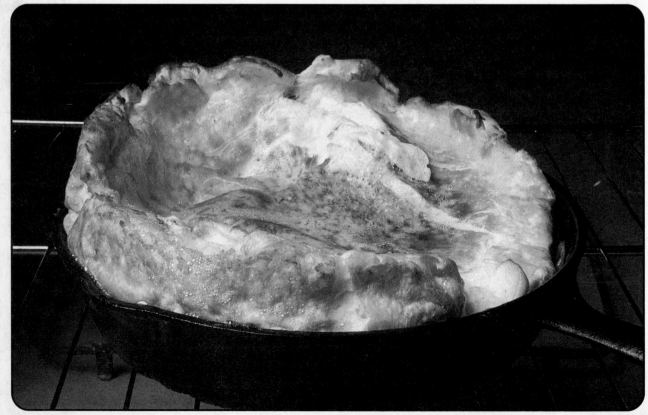

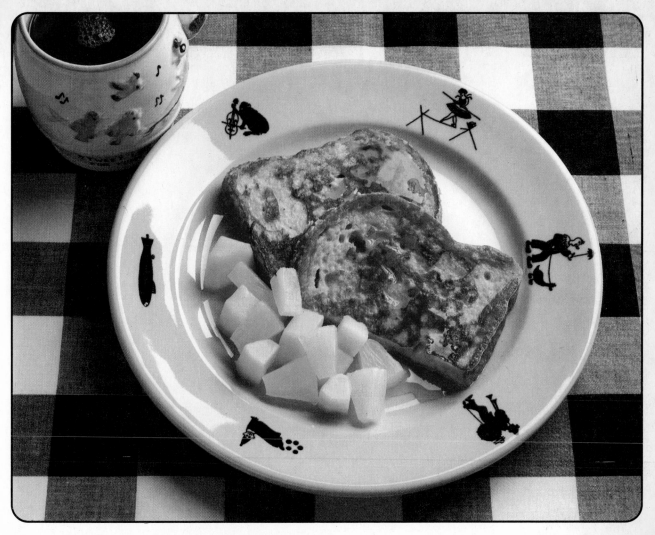

Banana French Toast

Serves 4

1 medium banana, mashed or pureed
2 eggs
⅓ cup low-fat or skim milk
⅛ tsp. ground mace
6 slices bread, each slice cut in half
1 tbsp. vegetable oil
1 tbsp. margarine or butter

- Beat the banana and the eggs together in a bowl.
- Stir in the milk and the mace.
- Dip the bread slices into the banana mixture, turning the bread to coat both sides.
- Heat the oil and the margarine or butter in a nonstick skillet over medium heat. When the margarine begins to foam, place the bread in the pan. Cook the french toast until it is well browned on both sides—about two minutes per side.
- Serve the french toast hot, accompanied by syrup and sliced fruit.

Sandwiches, Soups, and Snacks

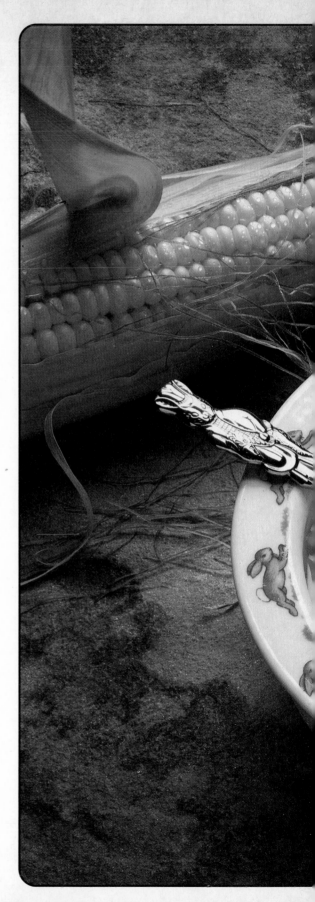

Corn-and-Potato Soup

Serves 4

1 small onion, grated
½ cup diced lean ham
2 tsp. vegetable oil
1 large potato, peeled and grated
3 cups reduced-sodium chicken broth
½ cup corn kernels, frozen or canned
⅛ tsp. pepper

- In a saucepan over medium-low heat, cook the onion and ham in the oil until the onion is transparent—about five minutes.
- Add the potato and chicken broth to the saucepan.
- Bring the soup to a simmer and cook until the potato is tender—about 20 minutes.
- Stir in the corn and the pepper and heat through.

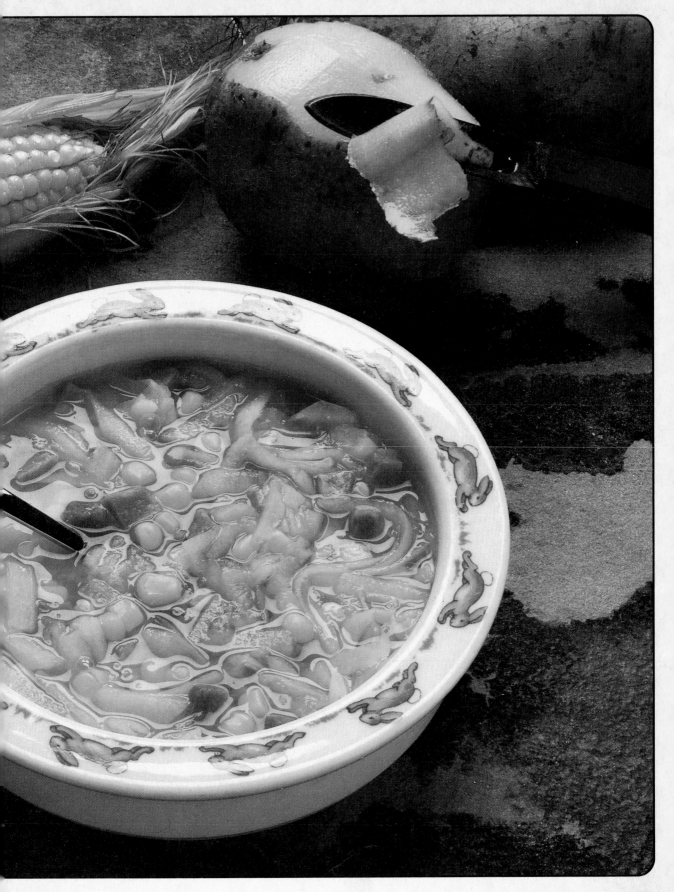

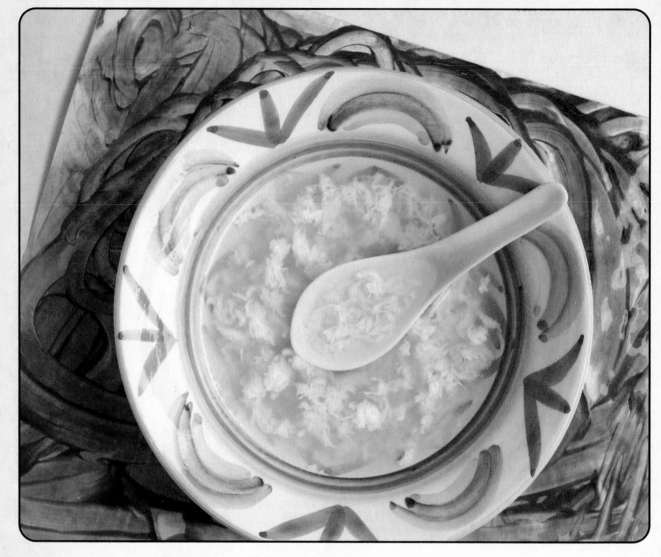

Egg Drop Soup with Rice

Serves 4

    4 cups reduced-sodium chicken broth
    1 cup cooked rice
    2 eggs, beaten
    lemon juice and pepper for seasoning (optional)

- Put the chicken broth and the rice in a saucepan and bring the mixture to a full boil.
- Stirring the broth constantly with a circular motion, slowly pour in the eggs.
- Taste the soup for seasoning: Add a little lemon juice and pepper, if desired. Serve hot.

Grilled Cheese Sandwiches with Pineapple and Canadian Bacon

Makes 4 sandwiches

8 slices whole-wheat bread
4 tsp. margarine or butter, softened
8 thin slices cheddar cheese
4 canned pineapple rings packed in juice, drained
4 thin slices Canadian bacon, any fat removed

- Spread ½ teaspoon of the margarine or butter on one side of each slice of bread. Place the slices buttered side down on a clean work surface.
- Top four of the bread slices with a slice of cheese, a pineapple ring, a slice of bacon, and another slice of cheese.
- Cover each sandwich with one of the remaining slices of bread, buttered side up.
- Place the sandwiches in a large nonstick skillet over low heat and grill them until they are nicely browned — about two minutes per side.

Chunky Tomato Soup with Cheesy Popcorn

Serves 4

one 10½-oz. can condensed tomato soup
1 cup low-fat or skim milk
1 large, ripe tomato, chopped
2 tbsp. unpopped popcorn kernels
3 tbsp. finely grated cheddar cheese
2 tbsp. finely grated Parmesan

- Combine the tomato soup, milk, and chopped tomato in a saucepan.
- Bring the soup to a simmer over medium heat, stirring occasionally, then reduce the heat to low to keep the soup warm while you make the popcorn.
- Pop the corn in a hot-air popper. While the popcorn is still hot, add the cheeses and toss the mixture well.
- Serve the soup hot and pass the popcorn.

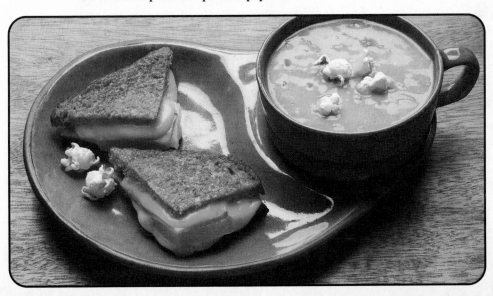

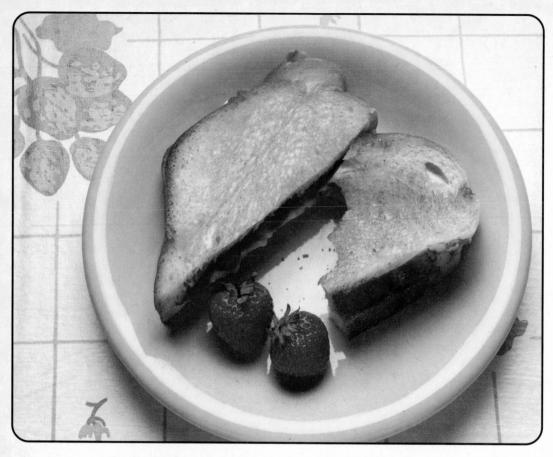

Grilled Ricotta-and-Jam Sandwiches

Makes 4 sandwiches

4 tsp. margarine or butter, softened
8 slices hallah or egg bread
4 tbsp. strawberry or raspberry jam
1½ cups part-skim ricotta cheese
1 cup fresh strawberries, raspberries, or other fresh fruit, for garnish

- Spread ½ teaspoon of the margarine or butter on one side of each slice of bread. Lay the slices buttered side down on a clean work surface.
- Spread 1 tablespoon of the jam onto the unbuttered side of four of the bread slices.
- Spread the ricotta cheese over the jam.
- Cover each sandwich with one of the remaining slices of bread, buttered side up.
- Cook the sandwiches in a large nonstick skillet over low heat, turning once, until they are evenly browned on both sides—about two minutes per side.
- When the sandwiches are cooked, cut them in half and garnish each one with some of the fruit.

116

Tuna-Carrot Salad Pita Pockets

Makes 4 sandwiches

   one 6½-oz. can water-packed white tuna, drained
   1 medium carrot, grated (about ¾ cup)
   ⅓ cup raisins
   2 tbsp. reduced-calorie mayonnaise
   ½ tsp. curry powder (optional)
   four 4-inch whole-wheat pita loaves
   4 lettuce leaves

- Combine the tuna, grated carrot, raisins, and mayonnaise. If you are using the curry powder, add it too.
- Slice a 1-inch piece from one side of each pita loaf to make it into a pocket.
- Stuff a lettuce leaf inside each pita loaf.
- Spoon a quarter of the tuna mixture into each sandwich.

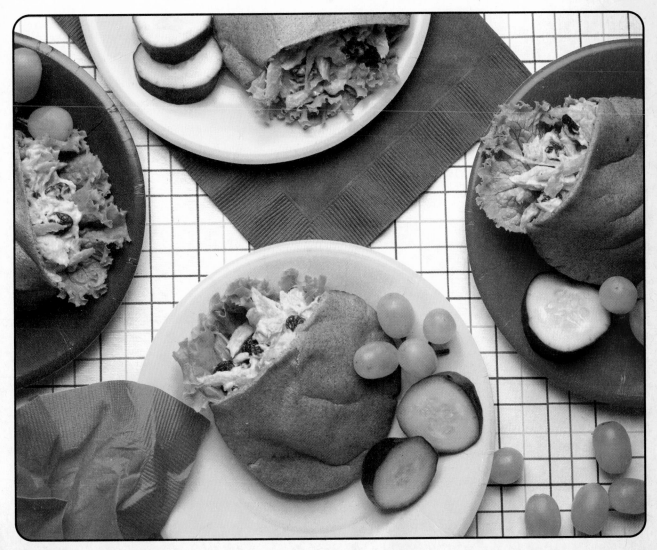

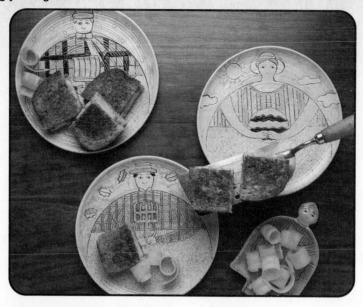

Grilled Peanut-Butter-and-Apple Sandwiches

Makes 4 sandwiches

> 4 tsp. margarine or butter, softened
> 8 slices whole-wheat bread
> ½ cup peanut butter
> 1 cup unsweetened canned apple slices, drained

- Spread ½ teaspoon of the margarine or butter on one side of each slice of bread. Place the slices buttered side down on a clean work surface.
- Spread 1 tablespoon of the peanut butter onto the unbuttered side of each slice of bread.
- Arrange one-quarter of the apple slices on a slice of bread. Repeat with the remaining apples and three more bread slices.
- Cover the apples with the remaining slices of bread, peanut butter sides down.
- Place the sandwiches in a large nonstick skillet over very low heat and grill them, turning once, until they are browned on both sides — about two minutes per side.

Turkey-Apple Salad Sandwiches

Makes 4 sandwiches

> ¾ cup diced cooked turkey (about ⅓ lb.)
> ¼ cup diced celery
> ½ cup diced apple
> ¼ cup reduced-calorie mayonnaise
> ⅓ cup chopped walnuts (optional)
> 4 whole-wheat english muffins
> 4 lettuce leaves

- Combine the turkey, celery, apple, mayonnaise, and the walnuts, if you are using them.
- Separate the english muffins with a fork or slice them in half horizontally and then toast them.
- Lay a lettuce leaf on top of each of four muffin halves. Spoon one-fourth of the turkey salad onto each lettuce leaf. Top each sandwich with the other muffin half.

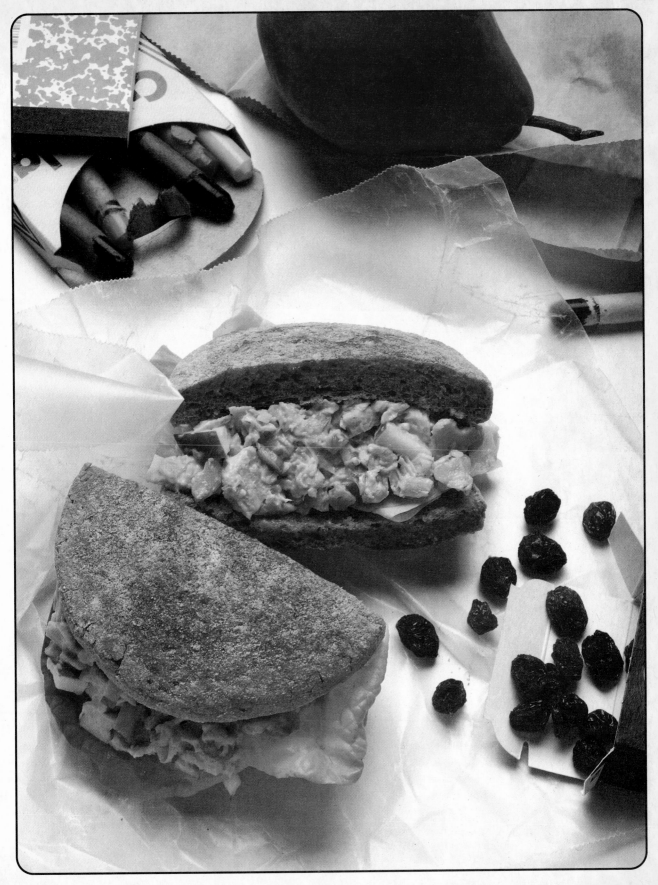

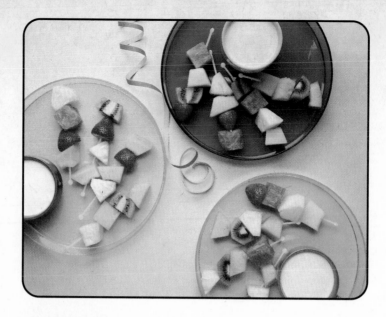

Fruit Dips

Strawberries, apples, grapes as well as peeled, chunked cantaloupe, pineapple, papaya, and banana all make fine fruits for dipping. For skewers, you will need 16 thin party sticks with blunt ends, such as swizzle sticks, each about 5 inches long.

Serves 4

64 fruit chunks, each about 1 inch wide

- Push a skewer through the centers of four mixed fruit chunks. Repeat with the remaining fruit and skewers.
- To serve, allow each person four skewers and let him dip the fruit into any of the following three dipping sauces.

Orange-Ricotta Dipping Sauce

½ cup part-skim ricotta
2 tbsp. orange-juice concentrate
½ tsp. vanilla extract
1 tsp. sugar

- Put all of the ingredients into a blender or a food processor and process them until they are smooth.

Maple-Yogurt Dipping Sauce

2 tbsp. plain low-fat yogurt
3 oz. light cream cheese
1 tbsp. maple syrup

- Put the yogurt, cream cheese, and maple syrup into a blender or a food processor and process them until they are smooth.

Raspberry Dipping Sauce

¼ cup light cream cheese
¼ cup vanilla low-fat yogurt
2 tbsp. fresh or frozen unsweetened raspberries

- Put the cream cheese, yogurt, and raspberries into a food processor or a blender and process them until they are smooth. Substitute raspberry jam or unsweetened fresh or frozen strawberries for the raspberries, if you wish.

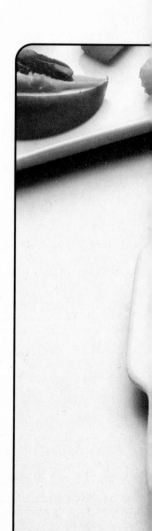

Garnished Celery, Apples, and Cucumber

Once the fruit and vegetables are cut, children can prepare this snack themselves.

Celery, cut into 2-inch lengths
Apples, unpeeled, cut into wedges and cored
Cucumbers, sliced into circles ¼ inch thick

For spreading:

Light cream cheese
Peanut butter
Cold-pack cheese spread

For sprinkling:

Chopped chives
Chopped dates, apricots, or other dried fruit
Bean Sprouts
Raisins
Chopped sunflower seeds
Chopped nuts
Granola

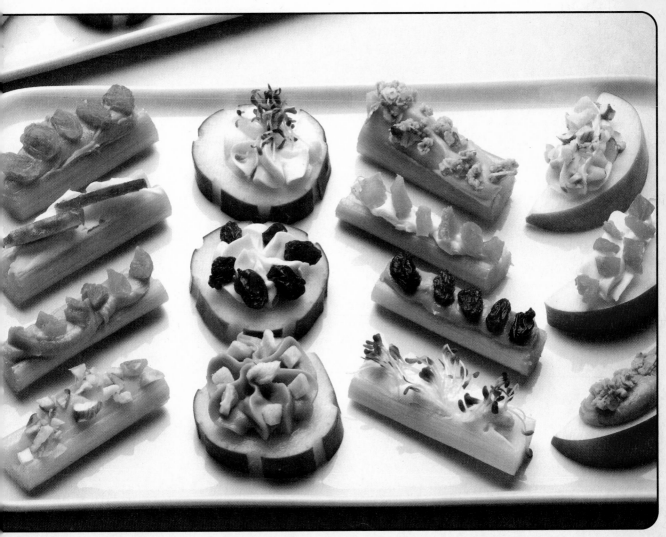

Main Dishes

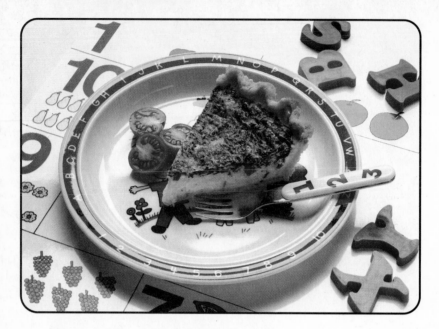

Three-Cheese Spinach Pie

Serves 8

> 1 cup grated part-skim mozzarella
> 1 cup grated Swiss cheese
> 1/2 cup grated Parmesan
> 1 deep 9-inch unbaked piecrust
> 4 eggs
> 2 cups low-fat or skim milk
> 1/4 tsp. grated nutmeg
> 1/4 cup chopped sweet red or green pepper
> 1/2 cup frozen chopped spinach, thawed and squeezed to remove excess moisture

- Preheat the oven to 350° F.
- Sprinkle the cheeses into the unbaked piecrust.
- Put the eggs, milk, and nutmeg in a bowl and whisk them together. Add the chopped pepper.
- Scatter the spinach over the cheeses in the piecrust.
- Carefully pour the egg mixture into the shell.
- Bake the pie until it is puffy and browned — about 45 minutes.

Corn Muffin Sloppy Joes

Both the corn muffins and the beef mixture can be made ahead of time and frozen.

Serves 4

Corn Muffins

> 1/2 cup all-purpose flour
> 1/4 cup yellow cornmeal
> 1 tbsp. sugar
> 1 tsp. baking powder
> 1 egg
> 1 1/2 tbsp. vegetable oil
> 1/2 cup buttermilk or plain low-fat yogurt

- Preheat the oven to 350° F.
- Line four muffin cups with paper or foil baking cups.
- Sift the flour, cornmeal, sugar, and baking powder together.
- Put the egg, oil, and buttermilk or yogurt in a bowl and whisk them until they are blended.
- Add the sifted ingredients to the egg mixture and stir just until the dry ingredients are blended in.
- Spoon the batter into the lined muffin cups.
- Bake the muffins until they have browned lightly on top—20 to 25 minutes.

Beef Mixture

½ lb. lean ground beef
½ cup canned kidney beans or pinto beans, drained and rinsed
1 cup mild taco sauce
1 cup canned unsalted whole tomatoes, chopped
½ tsp. chili powder
½ cup grated Monterey Jack or mild cheddar cheese
2 cups shredded lettuce or cabbage
4 tbsp. plain low-fat yogurt or half-and-half sour cream

- While the corn muffins *(recipe above)* are baking, make the beef mixture. First, fry the ground beef in a large skillet set over medium-low heat. As the meat cooks, break up the clumps; cook the beef until it loses all of its red color. Drain off the fat and discard it.
- Add the beans to the beef, along with the taco sauce, tomatoes, and chili powder. Simmer the mixture for 10 minutes.
- To serve the Sloppy Joes, slice each corn muffin in half horizontally. Spoon some of the Sloppy Joe mixture onto the bottom half of each muffin and top the mixture with the other half of the muffin.
- Put the grated cheese, lettuce or cabbage, and yogurt or sour cream in separate bowls and let the diners help themselves.

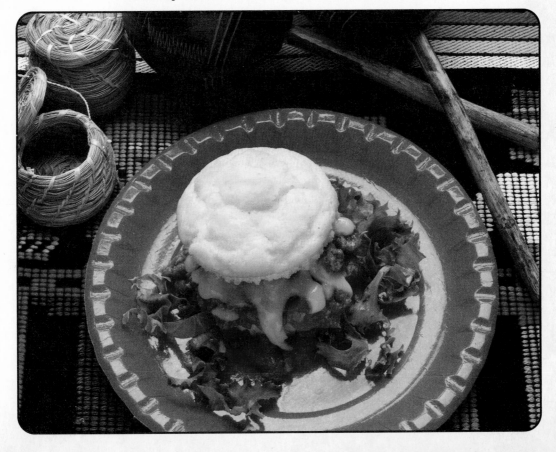

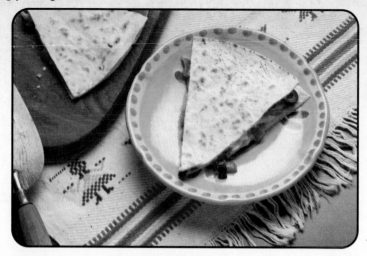

Vegetable Quesadillas

Serves 4

½ cup vegetarian refried beans
four 10-inch flour tortillas
½ cup grated Monterey Jack or mild cheddar cheese
8 black olives, sliced (optional)
¼ cup chopped sweet red or green pepper
2 small tomatoes, thinly sliced

- Spread the refried beans over two of the tortillas. Sprinkle half of the cheese over the beans, and if you are using the olives, spread them over the cheese. Scatter the chopped pepper over the cheese and then arrange the sliced tomatoes on top. Sprinkle the remaining cheese over the two quesadillas and top each one with a tortilla.
- Heat a large heavy-bottomed skillet over medium-high heat. Place one quesadilla in the skillet and cook it, turning once, until the cheese has melted and brown spots have formed on the tortillas—about two minutes. Transfer the cooked quesadilla to a cutting board and cook the remaining quesadilla the same way.
- Cut each quesadilla into six wedges before serving.

Chicken Tostados

Serves 4

2 to 3 tbsp. vegetable oil
four 6-inch corn tortillas
2 cups cooked shredded or slivered chicken
½ cup half-and-half sour cream
2 hard-boiled eggs, chopped
1 cup grated Monterey Jack or mild cheddar cheese
2 cups shredded lettuce or cabbage
1 large tomato, chopped
8 black olives, sliced (optional)
½ avocado, thinly sliced (optional)

- Set a heavy-bottomed skillet over medium-high heat and add enough vegetable oil to cover the bottom of the pan by ¼ inch. When the oil is hot, fry each tortilla until it is crisp—about 45 seconds. Drain the fried tortillas on paper towels.
- Put the chicken and the sour cream in a small saucepan over low heat and cook, stirring occasionally, until the mixture is heated through—about five minutes.
- To serve, give each person a tortilla and let him help himself to the chicken, eggs, cheese, lettuce, tomato, and, if you are using them, the olives and avocado.

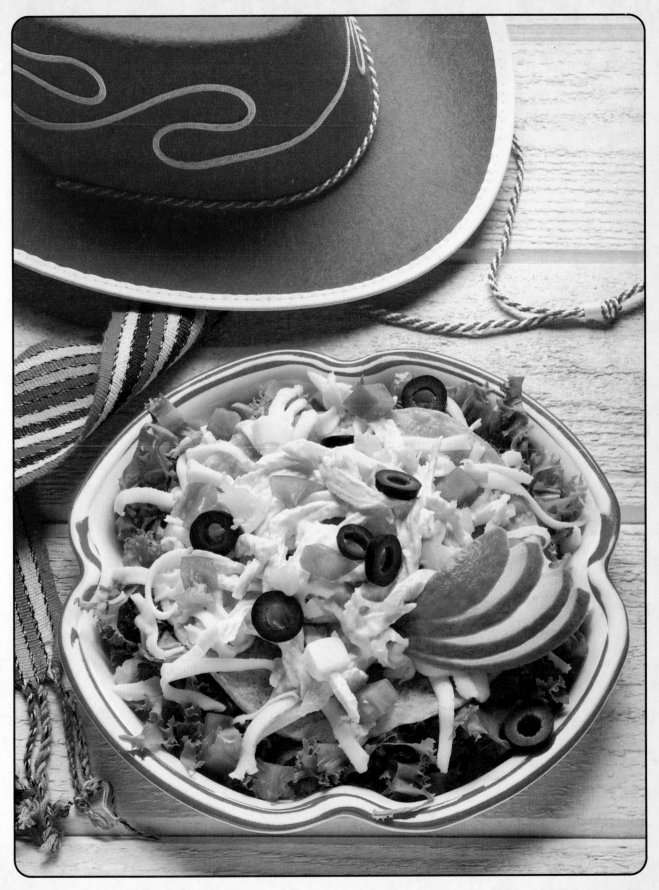

Pasta with Cheese and Ham

Serves 4

3 eggs, beaten
1 cup low-fat or skim milk
¾ cup grated Parmesan
freshly ground black pepper
2 tsp. salt
12 oz. fusilli (known also as rotini and spirals)
1 tbsp. margarine or butter
½ cup lean ham, sliced into short, narrow strips

- Bring 4 quarts of water to a boil.
- Put the eggs, milk, Parmesan, and a generous grinding of pepper into a bowl and whisk until they are blended.
- When the water is boiling, add the salt and the fusilli. Start testing the pasta after eight minutes and cook it until it is *al dente*. Drain the pasta and rinse it under cold running water to keep it from sticking. Set it aside.
- Lightly sauté the ham strips in a nonstick pan over medium heat until thoroughly warm, then set aside.
- In a large skillet over low heat, melt the margarine or butter. Pour the egg mixture into the skillet and cook it until the edges begin to set—about 30 seconds. Add the pasta and raise the heat to medium. Stirring constantly, cook the mixture until the pasta is very hot and the eggs have thickened, about four minutes.
- Serve the pasta with the ham scattered on top.

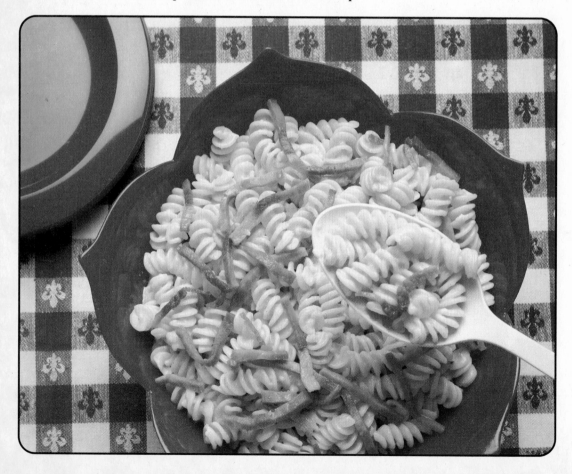

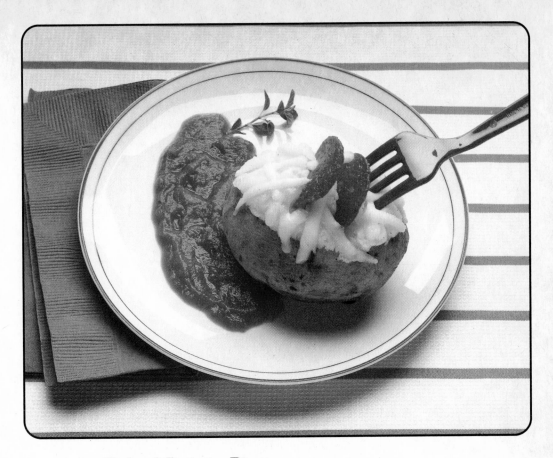

Baked Potato Pizza

Serves 4

4 large potatoes, baked
¾ cup grated part-skim mozzarella
½ cup grated Parmesan
½ cup low-fat or skim milk
¾ cup unsalted tomato sauce
8 thin slices pepperoni

- Preheat the oven to 350° F.
- Cut a slice from the side of each potato to create an opening about 1½ inches wide. Discard the potato slices or reserve them for another use.
- Scoop most of the flesh out of the potatoes; transfer the potato flesh to a bowl.
- Mash the potato flesh thoroughly with a potato masher or a fork.
- Add ½ cup of the mozzarella, the Parmesan, and the milk to the mashed potato and stir until well mixed.
- Pour a tablespoonful of the tomato sauce into each potato shell.
- Divide the mashed potato mixture among the four shells.
- Sprinkle 1 tablespoon of the remaining mozzarella onto each potato and place two slices of pepperoni on top.
- Put the potatoes on a baking sheet and bake them until the cheese has melted completely and the potatoes are very hot — about 30 minutes.
- Heat the remaining tomato sauce and serve it with the potatoes.

Fish Baked in Foil

Any firm, white-fleshed fish, such as snapper, hake, grouper, tilefish, or flounder, works well for this recipe.

Serves 6

2 medium potatoes, peeled and very thinly sliced
4 tsp. margarine or butter
four 4- to 6-oz. fish fillets, about ½ inch thick each
1 carrot, very thinly sliced
1/2 bunch chives, finely cut, or 2 or 3 green tops of scallions, finely chopped

- Preheat the oven to 400° F.
- Cut four 8-by-12-inch pieces of foil.
- Lay a piece of the foil on a clean work surface, shiny side up. Arrange one-fourth of the potato slices near the center of the foil. Put 1/2 teaspoon of the margarine or butter on top of the potato and lay a fish fillet on top of the margarine or butter. Sprinkle the fish with one fourth of the carrot slices and chives or scallions and put another 1/2 teaspoon of the margarine or butter on top. Fold the foil loosely, with the dull side out, and seal the edges so that the seams are tight, but there is still a pocket of air trapped inside. Repeat with the remaining foil and ingredients to form four packages.
- Put the packages on a baking sheet and bake them for 20 minutes. Fish that is very cold or thicker than ½ inch may take longer; check to make sure that the fish is opaque before serving it.

Note: These fish packages can also be cooked outdoors, directly on coals or on a grill. The wrapped fish will cook in less time if cooked directly on hot coals.

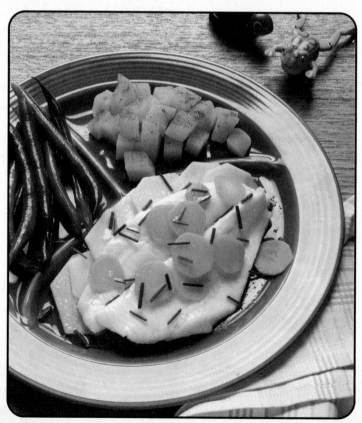

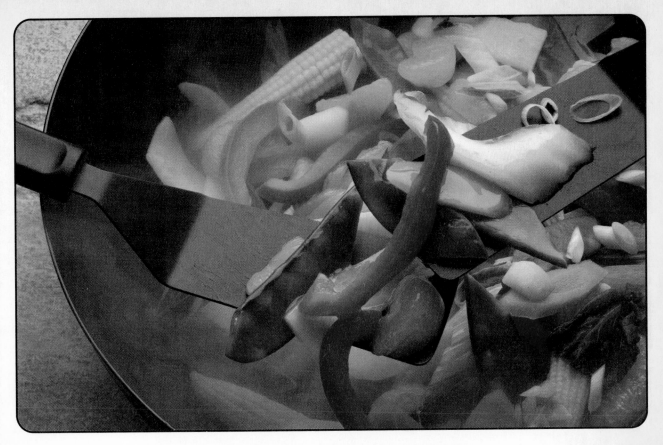

Mandarin Orange Vegetable Stir-Fry

Serve this colorful stir-fry with either rice or noodles.

Serves 4

½ cup orange-juice concentrate
1 tbsp. low-sodium soy sauce
2 tbsp. rice vinegar or white vinegar
1 tbsp. cornstarch
2 tbsp. vegetable oil
1 medium carrot, thinly sliced on the diagonal
1 red, green, or yellow pepper, seeded, deribbed, and thinly sliced
1 cup sliced bok choy or other cabbage
1 cup fresh or frozen snow peas
1 cup canned, drained mandarin oranges
½ cup canned, drained, sliced water chestnuts
½ cup canned, drained, sliced bamboo shoots (optional)
8 ears canned baby corn, split lengthwise (optional)
4 scallions (green onions), trimmed and thinly sliced on the diagonal
¼ cup toasted cashews (optional)

- In a small bowl, combine the orange-juice concentrate, soy sauce, vinegar, cornstarch, and ¼ cup water.
- Heat the oil in a wok or large nonstick skillet over high heat until it just begins to smoke. Add the carrot and stir-fry it for 15 seconds. Add the pepper and stir-fry for 30 seconds. Add the bok choy or cabbage, snow peas, oranges, water chestnuts, and the bamboo shoots and corn, if you are using them, and stir-fry the mixture for 30 seconds more.
- Add the cornstarch mixture and allow the liquid to come to a boil, stirring until the sauce thickens.
- Stir in the scallions just before serving, spoon the dish into a serving bowl, and then scatter the cashews on top, if you are using them.

Beverages

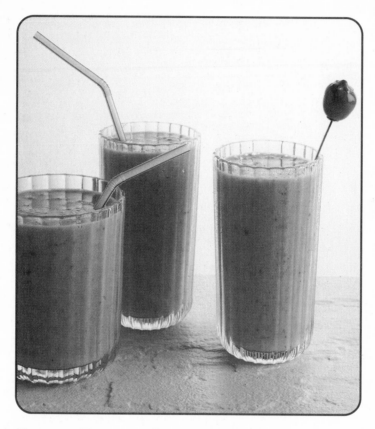

Frozen Banana-Strawberry Shake

Serves 2

1 banana, peeled, wrapped in plastic wrap and frozen
6 fresh or unsweetened frozen strawberries
¼ cup low-fat vanilla yogurt
1 tbsp. cranberry juice

- Cut the frozen banana into 2-inch lengths and put them into a blender or a food processor. Add the strawberries, yogurt, and cranberry juice.
- Process the mixture until it is smooth.
- Pour the shake into a glass and, if you like, serve it garnished with a whole strawberry.

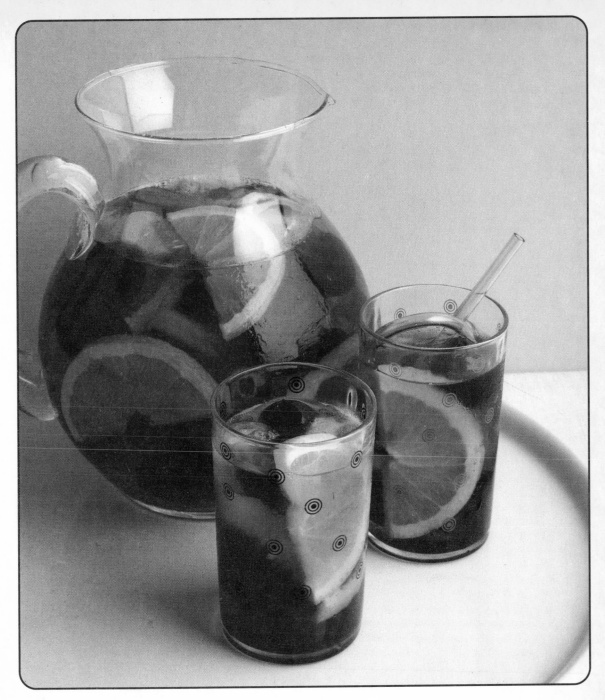

Fruit Fizz

Serves 4

1 cup apple juice
¼ cup limeade concentrate
½ cup cranberry juice
1 cup fresh or frozen cherries, pitted
1 large seedless orange, peeled, cut in half and sliced
1 cup sodium-free seltzer water

- In a pitcher, stir all ingredients but the seltzer together.
- Add the seltzer and stir.
- Pour this fruit fizz into tall glasses filled with plenty of ice. Serve, if you like, with a spoon.

Occasional Treats

The following special treats might be served as occasional after-school snacks or desserts to children. Although they are made with such wholesome ingredients as whole wheat flour, bran, and fruits, they contain fat. You will want, therefore, to serve them in moderation, perhaps saving them for days when the family menu has been particularly low in fat.

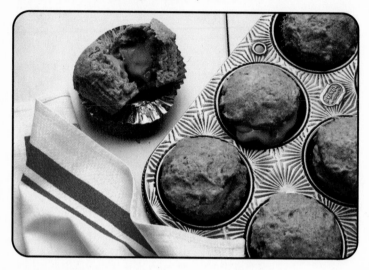

Surprise Banana-Bran Muffins

Makes 12 muffins

> 3 tbsp. margarine or butter
> 1/3 cup light brown sugar
> 1 cup bran cereal
> 2 or 3 ripe bananas, mashed (1 to 1½ cups)
> 1 egg
> 1½ cups all-purpose flour
> 1½ tsp. baking powder
> ¾ cup peanut butter

- Preheat the oven to 350° F.
- Line 12 muffin cups with paper or foil baking cups.
- Cream the margarine or butter with the sugar in a bowl.
- Stir in the bran cereal and the bananas.
- Mix in ¼ cup very hot water.
- Add the egg and beat it in.
- Sift in the flour and the baking powder. Stir just until the dry ingredients are mixed in; do not overmix.
- Drop a heaping tablespoonful of the batter into each lined cup. Drop a tablespoonful of the peanut butter onto the batter in each cup, using up all of the peanut butter. To cover up the peanut butter surprise, divide the remaining batter equally among the partially filled cups.
- Bake the banana-bran muffins until they are evenly browned — 20 to 25 minutes.

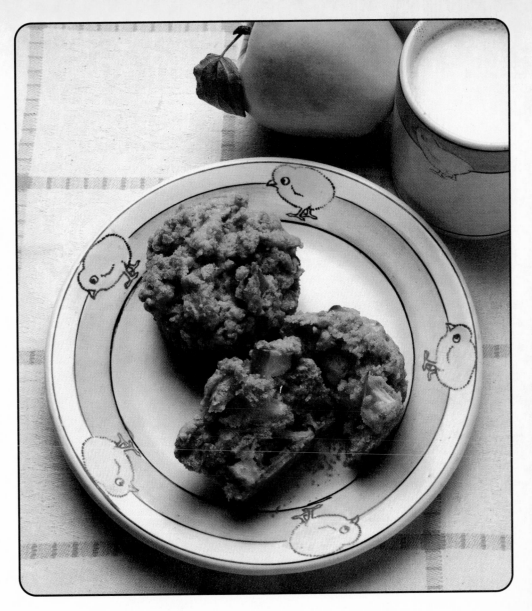

Fresh Apple Cupcakes

Makes 6 cupcakes

⅔ cup all-purpose flour
⅓ cup whole wheat flour
⅓ cup sugar
½ tsp. baking soda
½ tsp. ground ginger
⅓ cup vegetable oil
1 egg
1⅓ cup cored, chopped apple (unpeeled)
1 tsp. vanilla extract

● Preheat the oven to 350° F.
● Line six muffin cups with paper or foil baking cups.
● Sift the flours, sugar, baking soda, and ginger together into a bowl.
● Add the oil, egg, apple, and vanilla and stir just until all of the flour is mixed in.
● Divide the batter among the lined muffin cups.
● Bake the cupcakes until they are puffy and nicely browned — 35 to 40 minutes.

Cranberry-Pineapple Crunch

These individual desserts are delicious as they are, warm or cold, but they may also be served with a dollop of yogurt or a scoop of ice milk.

Serves 4

⅔ cup whole-berry cranberry sauce
⅔ cup unsweetened pineapple pieces, fresh or canned, drained
¾ cup rolled oats
2 tbsp. bran cereal
¼ cup light brown sugar
2 tbsp. margarine or butter

- Preheat the oven to 350° F.
- Combine the cranberry sauce and the pineapple in a bowl.
- In another bowl, mix the oats, bran cereal, and sugar.
- Use your fingers or a wooden spoon to rub the margarine or butter into the oatmeal mixture; the mixture will be crumbly.
- Divide half of the oatmeal mixture among four 8-ounce baking cups.
- Press the oatmeal crumbs into each of the cups.
- Spoon a portion of the cranberry-pineapple mixture into each cup, dividing the mixture among the cups.
- Sprinkle a quarter of the remaining oatmeal crumbs on top of each dessert.
- Bake the desserts until they are brown and bubbly on top — 30 to 45 minutes.

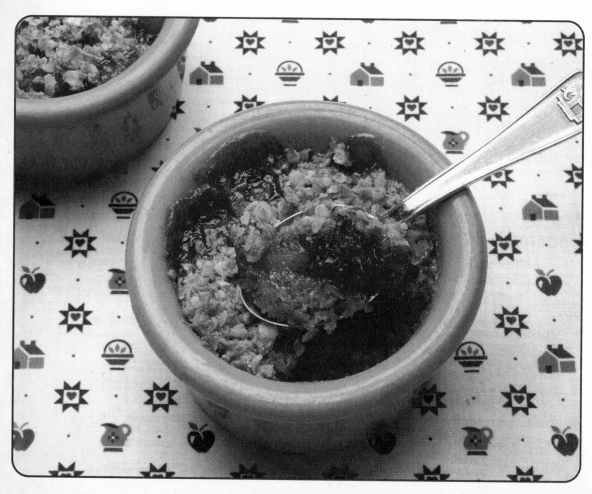

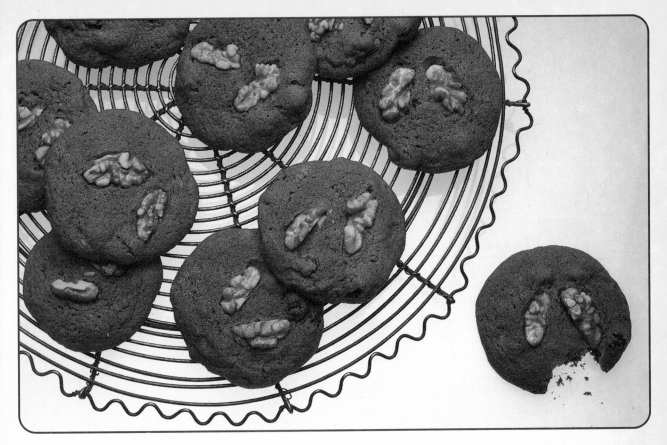

Cocoa Kiss Cookies

Makes 3 dozen cookies

½ cup margarine or butter
⅓ cup dark brown sugar
¼ cup white sugar
1 egg
1 cup all-purpose flour
½ cup whole wheat flour
½ tsp. baking soda
2 tbsp. unsweetened cocoa powder
½ cup raisins
⅓ cup walnut pieces (optional)

- Preheat the oven to 350° F.
- In a mixing bowl, cream the margarine or butter with the brown and white sugars.
- Beat in the egg.
- Sift the flours, baking soda, and cocoa into the bowl and stir the mixture until the dry ingredients are blended.
- Stir in the raisins.
- Drop the cookie dough by tablespoonfuls onto ungreased baking sheets, leaving about 2 inches between each cookie.
- If you are using the walnuts, lightly press a piece onto the top of each cookie.
- Bake the cookies until they are lightly browned but still slightly soft — eight to 10 minutes.

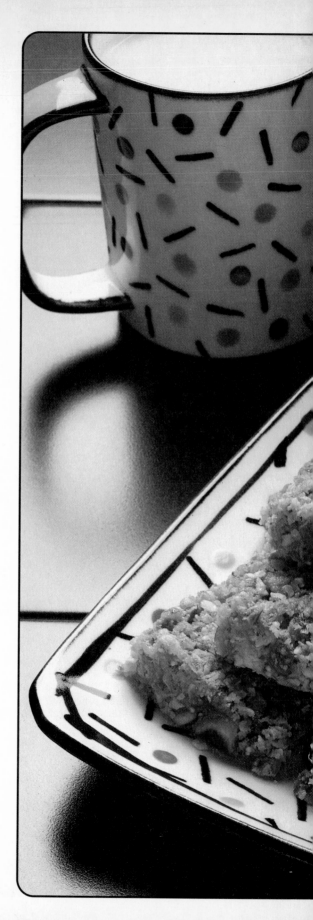

Figgy Oat Bars

Makes 45 bars

1 lb. dried figs, chopped
½ cup whole wheat flour
¼ cup all-purpose flour
¼ cup bran cereal
1 cup light brown sugar
1½ cups rolled oats
1 cup hazelnuts or whole unblanched almonds, finely chopped (optional)
1 cup margarine or butter, melted
2 tbsp. vegetable oil

- Preheat the oven to 350° F.
- In a bowl, combine the figs, flours, bran cereal, sugar, oats, and the nuts, if you are using them.
- Stir in the melted margarine or butter and the oil.
- Transfer the dough to a 10-by-15-inch jellyroll pan and use your fingers to spread it evenly on the pan.
- Bake the dough until the edges are brown — 25 to 30 minutes. Let the treat cool before cutting it into bars.

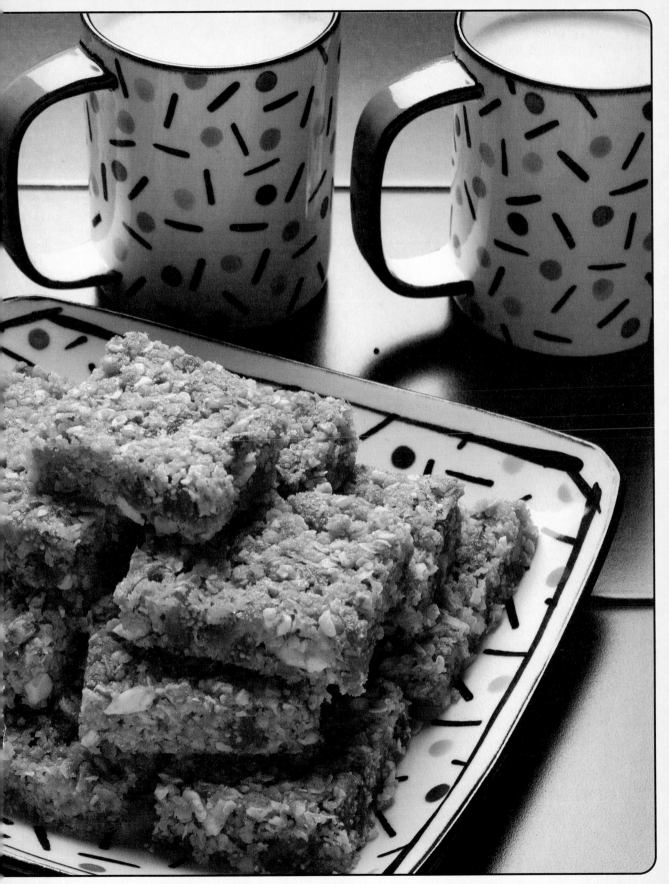

Bibliography

BOOKS

Ackerman, Caroline, *Cooking with Kids*. Mount Rainier, Md.: Gryphon House, 1981.

Akmakjian, Hiag, *The NATURAL Way to Raise a Healthy Child*. New York: Praeger, 1975.

Anderson, Linnea, et al., *Nutrition in Health and Disease*. Philadelphia: J. B. Lippincott, 1982.

Baker, Samm Sinclair, *The Indoor and Outdoor Grow-It Book*. New York: Random House, 1966.

Baker, Susan, M.D., *Parents' Guide to Nutrition*. Reading, Mass.: Addison-Wesley, 1986.

Behrman, Richard E., M.D., and Victor C. Vaughan III, M.D., *Nelson Textbook of Pediatrics*. Philadelphia: W. B. Saunders, 1983.

Boston Children's Medical Center and Richard I. Feinbloom, M.D., *Child Health Encyclopedia: The Complete Guide for Parents*. New York: Dell, 1975.

Brody, Jane, *Jane Brody's Nutrition Book*. New York: Bantam Books, 1982.

Cameron, Allan G., *Food — Facts and Fallacies*. London: Faber and Faber, 1971.

Carleton, R. Milton, *Indoor Gardening Fun: Year-Round Projects for Children*. Chicago: Reilly & Lee Books, 1970.

Castle, Sue:
The Complete New Guide to Preparing Baby Foods. Garden City, N.Y.: Doubleday, 1981.
Nutrition for Your Child's Most Important Years: Birth to Age Three. New York: Simon & Schuster, 1984.

Clarke-Stewart, Alison, and Susan Friedman, *Child Development: Infancy through Adolescence*. New York: John Wiley & Sons, 1987.

Cobb, Vicki, *Science Experiments You Can Eat*. Philadelphia: J. B. Lippincott, 1972.

Coffin, Lewis A., M.D., *Children's Nutrition: A Consumer's Guide*. Santa Barbara, Calif.: Capra Press, 1984.

Davis, John A., and John Dobbing, *Scientific Foundations of Paediatrics*. Philadelphia: W. B. Saunders, 1974.

DeLorenzo, Lorisa, and Robert John DeLorenzo, M.D., *Total Child Care: From Birth to Age Five*. Garden City, N.Y.: Doubleday, 1982.

de Villiers, S. J. A., and Eunice van der Berg, *Getting Ready to Cook*. Milwaukee: Gareth Stevens, 1983.

Dondiego, Barbara L., *Crafts for Kids: A Month-by-Month Idea Book*. Blue Ridge Summit, Pa.: Tab Books, 1984.

Faelten, Sharon, *The Complete Book of Minerals for Health*. Emmaus, Pa.: Rodale Press, 1981.

Faggella, Kathy, *Concept Cookery: Learning Concepts through Cooking*. Bridgeport, Conn.: First Teacher Press, 1985.

Ferreira, Nancy J., *The Mother-Child Cook Book*. Menlo Park, Calif.: Pacific Coast, 1969.

Firkaly, Susan Tate, *Into the Mouths of Babes*. White Hall, Va.: Betterway Publications, 1984.

Fomon, Samuel J., M.D., *Nutritional Disorders of Children: Prevention, Screening, and Followup*. Rockville, Md.: U.S. Department of Health, Education, and Welfare, 1978.

Forbes, Gilbert B., M.D., ed., *Pediatric Nutrition Handbook*. Elk Grove Village, Ill.: American Academy of Pediatrics, 1985.

Fryer, Lee, and Annette Dickinson, *A Dictionary of Food Supplements: A Guide for Buying Vitamins, Minerals, and Other Foods for Health*. New York: Mason/Charter, 1975.

Goodhart, Robert S., M.D., and Maurice E. Shils, M.D., *Modern Nutrition in Health and Disease*. Philadelphia: Lea & Febiger, 1980.

Goodwin, Mary T., and Gerry Pollen, *Creative Food Experiences for Children*. Washington, D.C.: Center for Science in the Public Interest, 1980.

Howard, Rosanne B., and Harland S. Winter, M.D., eds., *Nutrition and Feeding of Infants and Toddlers*. Boston: Little, Brown, 1984.

Ilg, Frances L., M.D., Louise Bates Ames, and Sidney M. Baker, M.D., *Child Behavior*. New York: Harper & Row, 1981.

Johnson, Thomas R., M.D., William M. Moore, M.D., and James E. Jeffries, eds., *Children Are Different: Developmental Physiology*. Columbus, Ohio: Ross Laboratories, 1978.

Kamen, Betty, and Si Kamen, *Kids Are What They Eat: What Every Parent Needs to Know about Nutrition*. New York: Arco, 1983.

La Leche League International, *The Womanly Art of Breastfeeding*. Franklin Park, Ill.: La Leche League International, 1981.

Lambert-Lagacé, Louise, *Feeding Your Child: From Infancy to Six Years Old*. New York: Beaufort Books, 1982.

Lansky, Vicki, *Feed Me! I'm Yours*. Deephaven, Minn.: Meadowbrook Press, 1981.

Leach, Penelope, *The Child Care Encyclopedia*. New York: Alfred A. Knopf, 1984.

Levine, Lois, *The Kids in the Kitchen Cookbook: How to Teach Your Child the Delights of Cooking and Eating*. New York: Macmillan, 1968.

Lorenzen, Evelyn J., M.D., ed., *Dietary Guidelines*. Houston, Tex.: Gulf, 1978.

McEntire, Patricia, *Mommy, I'm Hungry: How to Feed Your Child Nutritiously*. Sacramento, Calif.: Cougar Books, 1982.

McWilliams, Margaret, *Nutrition for the Growing Years*. New York: John Wiley & Sons, 1980.

Murdich, Jack, *Buying Produce*. New York: Hearst Books, 1986.

Osborn, Susan, ed., *The Great American Guide to Diet and Health*. New York: McGraw-Hill, 1982.

Packard, Vernal S., Jr., *Processed Foods and the Consumer: Additives, Labeling, Standards, and Nutrition*. Minneapolis: University of Minnesota Press, 1976.

Palmer, Sushma, and Shirley Ekvall, *Pediatric Nutrition in Developmental Disorders*. Springfield, Ill.: Charles C Thomas, 1978.

Parents' Nursery School, *Kids Are Natural Cooks*. Boston: Houghton Mifflin, 1974.

Peck, Leilani Brinkley, et al., *Focus on Food*. New York: McGraw-Hill, 1974.

Pipes, Peggy L., *Nutrition in Infancy and Childhood*. St. Louis: C. V. Mosby, 1981.

Rapp, Doris J., M.D., *Allergies & Your Family*. New York: Sterling, 1981.

Rudolph, Abraham M., M.D., ed., *Pediatrics*. Norwalk, Conn.: Appleton & Lange, 1987.

Samuels, Mike, M.D., and Nancy Samuels, *The Well Child Book*. New York: Summit Books, 1982.

Satter, Ellyn, *Child of Mine: Feeding with Love and Good Sense*. Palo Alto, Calif.: Bull, 1986.

Silberstein, Warren P., M.D., and Lawrence Galton, *Helping Your Child Grow Slim: Safe Dieting for Overweight Children and Adolescents*. New York: Simon and Schuster, 1982.

Speer, Frederic, M.D., *Food Allergy*. Boston: John Wright/PSG, 1983.

Stanway, Penny, and Andrew Stanway, *Breast Is Best: A Commonsense Approach to Breastfeeding*. Wauwatosa, Wis.: American Baby Books, 1978.

Staying Flexible: The Full Range of Motion, by the Editors of Time-Life Books (Fitness, Health & Nutrition series). Alexandria, Va.: Time-Life Books, 1987.

Stoppard, Miriam, *Day by Day Baby Care*. New York: Villard Books, 1983.

Tsang, Reginald C., and Buford Lee Nichols, Jr., M.D., eds., *Nutrition and Child Health: Perspectives for the 1980s*. New York: Alan R. Liss, 1981.

Turner, Mary Dustan, and James S. Turner, *Making Your Own Baby Food*. New York: Workman, 1976.

U.S. Department of Agriculture Yearbook 1979, *What's to Eat? And Other Questions Kids Ask about Foods*. Washington, D.C.: U.S. Department of Agriculture, 1979.

Wanamaker, Nancy, Kristin Hearn, and Sherrill Richarz, *More Than Graham Crackers: Nutrition Education & Food Preparation with Young Children*. Washington, D.C.: National Association for the Education of Young Children, 1984.

West, Richard, M.D., and Richard Dodds, M.D., *The Complete Medical Guide To Children's Ailments*. New York: Exeter Books, 1983.

Whitney, Eleanor Noss, and Corinne Balog Cataldo, *Understanding Normal and Clinical Nutrition*. St. Paul: West, 1983.

Wilkinson, J. F., *Don't Raise Your Child to Be a Fat Adult*. Indianapolis: Bobbs-Merrill, 1980.

Wilms, Barbara, *Crunchy Bananas and Other Great Recipes Kids Can Cook*. Salt Lake City: Falcon Books, 1984.

Winick, Myron, ed.:

Childhood Obesity. New York: John Wiley & Sons, 1975.

Nutritional Management of Genetic Disorders. New York: John Wiley & Sons, 1979.

Worth, Cecilia, *Breastfeeding Basics: Easy-to-Read, Easy-to-Use Directions for the Breast-feeding Mother*. New York: McGraw-Hill, 1983.

Wunderlich, Ray C., Jr., M.D., and Dwight K. Kalita, *Nourishing Your Child: A Bioecologic Approach*. New Canaan, Conn.: Keats, 1984.

Your Growing Child, by the Editors of Time-Life Books (Successful Parenting series). Alexandria, Va.: Time-Life Books, 1987.

PERIODICALS

Adkinson, N. Franklin, Jr., et al., "Immunology Outlook: Keeping Current on Allergic Reactions." *Patient Care*, November 30, 1983.

Birch, Leann Lipps, "Children's Food Preferences: Developmental Patterns and Environmental Influences." *Annals of Child Development*, Vol. 4, 1987.

Bock, S. Allan, M.D.:
"Food Sensitivity." *Nutrition News*, October 1984.
"Food Sensitivity: A Practical Approach." *Nutrition & the M.D.*, December 1982.

"Prospective Appraisal of Complaints of Adverse Reactions to Foods in Children during the First 3 Years of Life." *Pediatrics*, May 1987.

Butkus, Sue Nicholson, and L. Kathleen Mahan, "Food Allergies: Immunological Reactions to Food." *Journal of the American Dietetic Association*, May 1986.

Copeland, Linda, M.D., "Pediatricians' Reported Practices in the Assessment and Treatment of Attention Deficit Disorders." *Journal of Developmental and Behavioral Pediatrics*, August 1987.

Friedlander, Lynne, "Toddlers & Food — The Two Seldom Mix." *Mothers Today*, January/February 1984.

Garred, Eileen, "Is Breast Really Best?" *American Health*, October 1987.

Greenberg, Elisabeth, "Starting Early with Kids in the Kitchen." *Washington Post*, September 19, 1984.

Hamill, Peter V. V., et al., "NCHS Growth Charts, 1976." *Monthly Vital Statistics Report*, June 22, 1976.

Leinhas, Judith L., Cynthia C. McCaskill, and Hugh A. Sampson, "Food Allergy Challenges: Guidelines and Implications." *Journal of the American Dietetic Association*, May 1987.

Liebman, Bonnie F., "Eating for Two." *Nutrition*

Action: Health Letter, April 1987.

Loomis, Christine, "Santa's Helpers." *Parents,* November 1985.

Mindell, Earl, "Unsafe Food: How to Spot It, How to Prevent It." *Family Circle*, April 14, 1987.

Satter, Ellyn, "Relating Research to Practice." *Nutrition News*, February 1987.

OTHER PUBLICATIONS

American Heart Association, "The American Heart Association Diet: An Eating Plan for Healthy Americans." Dallas: American Heart Assoc., 1985.

Caplan, Frank, ed., "Ages and Stages Toy List." *Parents' Yellow Pages: A Directory by the Princeton Center for Infancy*, no date.

"Food Allergy." Washington, D.C.: Asthma & Allergy Foundation of America, no date.

"How to Buy Beef Roasts." Home and Garden Bulletin No. 146. Washington, D.C.: U.S. Department of Agriculture, June 1982.

"How to Buy Beef Steaks." Home and Garden Bulletin No. 145. Washington, D.C.: U.S. Department of Agriculture, June 1977.

"Meat and Poultry Labels Wrap It Up . . . With What You Need to Know." Home and Garden Bulletin No. 238. Washington, D.C.: U.S. Department of Agriculture, March 1987.

Acknowledgments and Picture Credits

The index for this book was prepared by Louise Hedberg. The editors also thank: Barbara Anderson, Human Nutrition Information Service, U.S. Department of Agriculture, Washington, D.C.; Sharon Conner, Bethesda, Md.; Libby Hamilton, Alexandria Hospital Library, Alexandria, Va.; Nancy Lendved, Washington, D.C.

The sources for the photographs in this book are listed below, followed by the sources for the illustrations. Credits from left to right are separated by semicolons; credits from top to bottom are separated by dashes.

Photographs. Cover: Roger Foley. 7-12: Roger Foley. 13: Suzanne Szasz—N. Mareschal/The Image Bank; Suzanne Szasz—Roger Foley (2). 14: Roger Foley. 15: Roger Foley—Susie Fitzhugh. 16-17: Roger Foley. 19: Susie Fitzhugh. 26: Nancy Blackwelder. 37: Beecie Kupersmith. 39-44: Larry Sherer. 55: Cynthia Foster. 65: Roger Foley. 83: Pat Lanza Field. 99: Cynthia Foster. 101: Aldo Tutino. 107-137: Reneé Comet.

Illustrations. 8-9: Kathe Scherr from photos by Beecie Kupersmith. 20-21: Kathe Scherr from photos by

Kathy Zinsmeister Price. 22: Kathe Scherr from photo by Marilyn Segall. 24: Kathe Scherr from photo by Beecie Kupersmith. 28-30: Donald Gates from photos by Beecie Kupersmith. 31: Donald Gates, center illustration from photo by Beecie Kupersmith. 32-35: Kathe Scherr from photos by Kathy Zinsmeister Price. 38: Lisa Semerad from photo by Susie Fitzhugh. 45: Lisa Semerad from photo by Beecie Kupersmith. 51: Lisa Semerad from photos by Reneé Comet. 52-53: Lisa Semerad from photos by Beecie Kupersmith. 58: Lisa Semerad from photo by Marion F. Briggs. 61: Lisa Semerad from photo by Marilyn Segall. 67-77: Elizabeth Wolf from photos by Beecie Kupersmith. 78-79: William Hennessy, Jr. 81: Elizabeth Wolf from photo by Beecie Kupersmith. 84-92: Marguerite E. Bell from photos by Beecie Kupersmith. 93: Marguerite E. Bell, bottom illustration from photo by Marion F. Briggs. 95: Marguerite E. Bell from photos by Beecie Kupersmith. 96: Marguerite E. Bell from photos by Neil Kagan; Beecie Kupersmith (2)—Marion F. Briggs; Beecie Kupersmith; Marion F. Briggs. 97: Marguerite E. Bell from photos by Beecie Kupersmith. 104: Elizabeth Wolf from photo by Beecie Kupersmith.

Props: 107: pottery, Martin's of Georgetown,

Washington, D.C. 108-109: handmade pottery, Mary George Kronstadt, Washington, D.C. 112-113: bowl, Christ Child Opportunity Shop, Washington, D.C.; spoon, Nancy Brucks, Washington, D.C. 114: bowl, Preferred Stock, Washington, D.C.; placemat, artwork by Alison and Stephanie Newman, Alexandria, Va. 116, 117: tablecloths, J.R. Yeager, Washington, D.C. 118: plates, Little Caledonia, Washington, D.C. 120-121: rectangular trays, Williams-Sonoma, Washington, D.C. 122: plate, Nancy Brucks, Washington, D.C.; placemat, Tree Top Toys, Inc., Washington, D.C. 123: cloth, baskets, and maracas, Guatemala House, Washington, D.C. 124: plate, Little Caledonia, Washington, D.C. 125: belt, Guatemala House, Washington, D.C. 127: plate, Martin's of Georgetown, Washington, D.C. 128: plate, Homeworks, Washington, D.C. 130: glasses, Kathy Swekel, Arnold, Md. 131: glasses, Tracy Samuel, Takoma Park, Md.; tray, Williams-Sonoma, Washington, D.C. 132: muffin tin, Mary Lynn Skutley, Washington, D.C. 133: pottery, Le Rez de Chaussée at Chenonceau Antiques, Washington, D.C. 134: spoon, Shirley Cherkasky, Alexandria, Va. 136-137: handmade porcelain, Dorothy Hafner, New York, N.Y.

Index

Time-Life Books Inc. offers a wide range of fine record-
ings, including a *Rock 'n' Roll Era* series. For subscription
information, call 1-800-621-7026 or write TIME-LIFE
MUSIC, P.O. Box C-32068, Richmond, Virginia 23261-2068.